Implementing Research
in the Clinical Setting

Implementing Research in the Clinical Setting

Edited by

CHRIS BASSETT BA(Hons), RN, RNT
Lecturer in Nursing, University of Sheffield

W
WHURR PUBLISHERS
LONDON AND PHILADELPHIA

© 2001 Whurr Publishers Ltd
First published 2001
by Whurr Publishers Ltd
19b Compton Terrace, London N1 2UN England and
325 Chestnut Street, Philadelphia PA 19106 USA

Reprinted 2002

British Library Cataloguing in Publication Data

A catalogue record for this book
is available from the British Library.

ISBN 1 86156 284 5

Contents

Contributors

Lorraine B ELLIS PhD, MSc, BA(Hons), RNT, RGN, CertEd, Lecturer in Nursing, University of Sheffield

Jane HADDOCK MMedSci, BSc(Hons), RGN, DPS(Nursing), Practice Development Adviser, Chesterfield and North Derbyshire Royal Hospital

Sue HOPKINS RGN, MMedSci, RNT, CHSM ONC, Head of Student Support, Central Sheffield University Hospitals

Mark LIMB PhD, BSc(Hons), RGN, RNT, Lecturer in Nursing, University of Sheffield

Gene W MARSH PhD, RN, Professor of Acute and Critical Care Nursing, University of Sheffield

Tracey MOORE MSc, BSc(Hons), RGN, PGDipEd, Lecturer in Nursing, University of Sheffield

To my big sister Pauline,
for her encouragement and interest over the years

Preface

One of the greatest health challenges of the 21st century for nurses and healthcare professionals alike is the successful and widespread implementation of valid and relevant research into real-world healthcare practice. For too long, healthcare researchers have laboured to produce seemingly endless and often high-quality research studies and reports, which unfortunately have, for the most part (for many of the reasons explored in this book), ended up unread and unused in the journals on dusty shelves in hospital and university libraries. Now at last academics, healthcare practitioners and the government have woken up to the fact that if we really are serious about improving the care and treatment we give our patients, we need to address this vital issue as a matter of urgency.

That is what this book is all about, getting research into practice. It is written to help provide the hard-working and dedicated healthcare professionals at the sharp end of care with hints, insights and really practical ways of implementing research into practice. I wish you well with this absolutely vital task!

Chris Bassett
March 2001

CHAPTER ONE

The importance of research in nursing practice

CHRIS BASSETT AND SUE HOPKINS

Introduction

Current, valid and reliable research is becoming more and more important to modern healthcare practice. The expectations of patients and their families are increasing, and they, quite rightly, expect their medical and nursing care to be the very best available. This book has been written to explore the key issues related to the implementation of research in practice.

There are many books that systematically investigate different types of research methodology; some touch on the difficulties of implementation, but few spend any real time considering the specific difficulties of implementing valid research in the clinical setting. This book is designed to help busy nurses, or indeed any healthcare professional, to get research into practice, which is a vital, but unfortunately generally neglected part of the research process. The book is written by nurses, who have experience in both undertaking research and implementing it in practice, in understandable language, which is as jargon-free as possible. It uses practical situations to illustrate some of the issues and offers practical advice throughout. There are also a series of reflective questions (Action points) to help you structure your learning needs and action plans for change. You do not of course need to do them if you do not want to.

The nurse and research

Nursing has certainly come a long way in the past few years. The role of the nurse has changed hugely; he or she now nurses in a wide variety of different environments, sometimes isolated from other colleagues. He or she may work in the community setting, for example, or as a nurse specialist, caring for patients and prescribing care and medication with a large measure of autonomy. Indeed, specialisation has become an integral part of modern nursing. With this trend has come the absolute requirement that nursing knowledge must be the best and most current available.

The nurse's responsibilities have changed and increased in conjunction with the expansion of the nurse's role. Patients and their families now, quite rightly, expect the nurse to have the answers and to practise in an efficient, safe and effective way. With this expectation, comes the the risk that if the nurse does not provide research-based care, the patient or family is increasingly likely to call the nurse to account. This may be through the hospital or community trust's complaints mechanism, via the United Kingdom Central Council's (UKCC) professional conduct committee or, ultimately, through the legal system and courts.

In line with these changes, education of nurses has begun to change quite drastically. It is now fully university-based and is becoming much more rigorous in its approach to the teaching of research. A major part of the nurse's role now includes the use of evidence-based practice to underpin the care and treatment he or she dispenses. Over the past 30 years or so in the UK, there has been a growing effort made in nursing towards research-based practice and this has helped, at least in part, to establish nursing as a true profession. This growing professional concern with the best-quality care has matched increasing governmental directives for evidence-based practice to become the norm. Research is seen by all as essential for improving and developing nursing care, aiding the evaluation of care and providing clearer guidelines for practice. This is clearly beneficial to the National Health Service (NHS) and, of course, to the patient.

Up-to-date information and research can be used to change practice, enhance clinical care and assist in the reorganisation of care in the rapidly changing world of healthcare. As well as the changes to pre-registration nurse education, there has been an increase in the provision of continuing education for qualified nurses. This is due, in part at least, to the implementation of the Post-Registration, Education and Practice scheme (PREP) introduced by the UKCC. Many nurses are also working towards higher academic qualifications, such as diplomas and degrees. Research-awareness modules are an integral part of all these courses.

> **Action point**
> - Take some time to think about how you feel about research in nursing.
> - Do you use it in your job regularly?
> - Do you feel at ease with it?
> - Do you think you know enough about research?
> - What are you going to do about it?

Research in healthcare

Until recently, the nursing profession in general has not placed a great deal of importance on research. Indeed, comparatively little nursing research has been undertaken in Britain and even less has been implemented. Practice has been based predominantly on historical approaches to care rather than following clear evidence of good practice. In recent years, however, there has been a refocusing on the need for research in the light of several government reports and statements made by academics relating to research:

- 'Nursing MUST become a research-based profession' was stated as long ago as 1972 in the Report of the Committee on Nursing (Briggs Report).
- 'Research is a way of thinking. It demands a critical approach to knowledge, an ability to formulate relevant questions and to search for answers' (Greenwood 1984).
- In *Every Nurse's Business* came the statement that 'The most important issue for research and development is to enhance the capability of all nurses to contribute to research and development both locally and nationally' (Trent Regional Health Authority 1993).

Research-based nursing practice is of vital importance for nursing today, and will, if supported, allow nurses and midwives to practise competently and with confidence. All nurses and midwives in hospitals, the community and the private sector must utilise research in all areas of practice in accordance with their requirement for accountability and responsibility (UKCC 1986). Research findings offer the nursing profession opportunities to enhance nursing care while expanding the body of nursing knowledge. This will certainly help nursing and midwifery to maintain and enhance the vital role it has in modern healthcare. The widespread introduction and use of research will, we believe, be one of the most important factors in the new era of nursing. This book has been written with this in mind, and is designed to provide the reader with the necessary background knowledge to understand better the research process. It is also written in such a way as to provide the nurse or healthcare professional with a great many practical suggestions and guidelines on how research-based practice may be implemented successfully in the clinical area.

The meaning of research in healthcare

The aim of research is to establish what best practice should be by producing evidence. Development is concerned with the planned, systematic introduction of research into healthcare practice by changing current practice if required. The research or audit process may help healthcare professionals identify the need for such developments.

Introducing change: the case for research

As highlighted above, the implementation of evidence-based care into clinical nursing practice has long been recognised as an important issue (Bassett 1995). However, the nursing profession is still struggling to base practice developments on research findings (Hunt 1981; Greenwood 1984; Lobiondo-Wood 1986).

The Department of Health document *Report of the Taskforce on the Strategy for Research in Nursing, Midwifery and Health Visiting* (DoH 1993b) stresses the need for research-based practice to become the common practice. Other authors have highlighted the benefits of this in terms of improved care with increased patient satisfaction. But despite the clear advantages reported in many papers, research-based practice is not as widespread as one might hope. In addition, there is a clear requirement for those working within NHS trusts and primary care groups (PCGs) to put the growing number of healthcare policies, such as *Health of the Nation* (DoH 1992), *A Vision for the Future* (DoH 1993a) and *Working in Partnership* (DoH 1994a), into action. British healthcare and nursing have not begun to meet the requirements described in these policies and this has led to the presence of not only a 'theory/practice' gap, but also a 'policy/practice gap' (Cutcliffe and Bassett 1997).

Auditing healthcare outcomes

In the context of health and illness, outcome is usually defined in terms of the achievement of or failure to achieve desired goals (Delamothe 1995).

Audit concerns the monitoring of current practice against standards, preferably employing criteria derived from research findings on best practice in addition to professional and management judgement and consumer preference. The relationship between research and practice is dynamic: research findings inform practice and practitioners inform research by identification of issues to be investigated. Not all nurses are required to undertake research – this would be unfeasible, because if they did, who would be left to look after the patients? However, all nurses should have the knowledge to become involved in the utilisation of valid research findings in their practice. As stated above, all nurses should have research awareness. Recommendations from the DoH (1994a) state that all nurses/midwives have a responsibility to be aware of research. There is, therefore, the expectation that all nurses will do the following.

> **Action point**
> * Question and critically evaluate current professional practice.
> * Keep up-to-date with research-based knowledge in their clinical field and utilise where appropriate.
> * Protect the rights of patients who have agreed to participate in research.
> * Do you do all of the above?

Research appreciation

This factor is considered to be a natural progression from research awareness. It is here that the nurse's questioning attitude is channelled into finding out how research is carried out. Many nurses and midwives have undertaken research appreciation courses, often as part of a diploma, degree or master's programme of pre- or post-basic education.

Appreciation involves:

- the critical analysis of research findings
- understanding methodologies
- being familiar with the research process
- influencing colleagues in the use of research data
- developing responsibility for one's own professional development in research.

As part of the strategy of increasing research usage in practice, we need to foster those who want to be involved in research. This will help ensure that resources are made available to meet each nurse's future educational needs regarding research awareness and application training.

Research application

If managed carefully this aspect of research can really make a difference to the nurse's daily practice. It can have the following benefits:

- Increased knowledge of illness, treatment and care leading to competent care and direct benefit to patients.
- Clearer more timely identification of effective resource management.
- Research utilisation raising the profile of nurses and midwives and promoting the status of the profession.

Differing approaches to research

Different types of research methodology can be used to enhance practice; these will be touched on throughout the book. Quantitative research underpins certain types of practice, whereas the application of social science research with a qualitative approach encourages a holistic, humanistic approach to patient care. The number of nurses and midwives presently engaged in research application is growing but it needs to be quantified to ensure resources are available for future educational needs.

Research ability

Healthcare technology assessment is an area of increasing importance to every nurse. Used in the widest possible sense, it refers to techniques, drugs, equipment and procedures used by healthcare professionals in the delivery of healthcare and rehabilitation to individuals, and the systems within which such care is delivered. It denotes any processes involving safety, efficacy, feasibility, indications for use, cost and cost-effectiveness, as well as social, economic and ethical consequences of care.

For nurses and midwives this may involve any or all of the following:

- The assessment of health technologies as part of routine practice and also in major clinical trials.
- Projects undertaken as part of a post-registration course.
- Action research: review and replication of previous studies.
- Nurses and midwives assisting medical staff in clinical trials.

Purchasers' requirements

Users and purchasers of healthcare services, e.g. PCGs, will also have their own requirements relating to research in the trusts, including:

- proof of research and audit
- evaluation of practice within the contracting process
- evidence of outcomes.

The drive for research in nursing and healthcare

Nursing as a profession has come to acknowledge the requirement to develop its own body of knowledge to meet the fast-changing healthcare needs of society. Practice is not consistently based on sound empirical evidence; we need well-researched evidence to help evaluate care given and, ultimately, change practice for the benefit of patients. Knowledge must also be continuously updated to take account of changes in policy, new technologies, changes in disease processes and increased public awareness.

Why do we need research?

If nursing is to be considered as a profession, it must continue to develop a distinct body of knowledge. We need to continually update our knowledge to ensure effective, safe, high-quality care. This is a professional obligation. We have to be able to justify and be accountable for the care we give, and be confident that it is the best care based on the best possible evidence currently available.

Nurse managers now have a clear responsibility to raise research awareness and appreciation in their staff, helping them create an environment conducive to the critical examination of current practice. A culture of 'valuing research' is vital to the application of research to practice. Management and education practice should also be based on valid research findings. The introduction of a purchaser-provider split in healthcare provision means healthcare professionals must demonstrate that care is clinically sound and cost-effective. Evidence-based practice demands that nurses examine their practices in all spheres, evaluate care and ensure that best possible evidence is disseminated as widely as possible.

Theory/practice gap

Action point

- Do you know of the theory/practice gap?
- Do you know what it means?
- Can you think of any practices that you carry out for your patients that could possibly be enhanced by a sounder research base?

The theory/practice gap is by no means a new phenomenon; it has been identified as existing in healthcare practice for many years. Recent powerful moves in the UK, both professionally and politically, to provide evidence-based practice have highlighted the gap, making it more visible. This factor has forced researchers to remember who their audience is, and to ensure that implementation is made part of the research process rather than being a separate process. Their role must no longer be to keep producing more and more research, but to have in their minds when they publish their findings the ways in which they can help implement it. As well as producing high-quality, valid and reliable research they must help people make decisions and assist their judgement in implementing the findings. They must remember that nurses are often unaware of research findings, may lack critical appraisal skills and may not have the time available to fully implement the research findings. The theory/practice gap exists as a result of the constraints on nurses who may find it difficult to access the, sometimes exclusive, world of research due to their already punishing commitments and lack of research preparation.

It is widely accepted within the UK's nursing community that a theory/practice gap exists. It is also questionable whether the integration of research into practice has been a success, and unfortunately something of a divide and a certain suspicion has evolved between those who produce research and those who are asked to use it. We all need to work to overcome this for the benefit of our patients.

Conflicts and solutions: the future of the theory/practice gap

When the theory/practice gap is discussed there is a tendency for nurses to think of theory and practice as separate endeavours. Nurses in practice and nurse educators have tended to focus on how to achieve greater theory/practice integration.

Carr (1986) developed an approach using four factors to help link educational theory with the theory/practice gap. In his model, he considered the following factors:

- The 'applied science approach': helping relate theory as objective evidence, used to guide and regulate practice.
- The 'common-sense approach': identifying theory as being within the collective understanding of practitioners. Theory can be extracted from 'good' practice. This is an example of theory actually being 'driven' by practice.

- The 'practice approach': identifies theory as being knowledge derived from practical activities, which can then be used to guide decision making. There is also the belief that the nurse has a moral commitment to 'good' practice.
- The 'critical approach': brings together 'applied science' and 'practical' approaches of care. Theory, therefore, is derived by nurses gaining further insight into practice, increasing their autonomy.

Theory and practice can work in both directions: theory informs practice and practice helps to develop theory. Theory and practice can be considered as quite distinct; it becomes clear that if the two are not used in conjunction, research-based nursing may not occur. This therefore makes the assumption that a gap does exist and that there are ways of reducing this gap. Theory is what is taught in school, practice is what happens on the wards and in the community; the theorist, usually perceived as an educator or researcher, and the practitioner are seen as different and separate beings (Ellis 1992).

The reality is that practising nurses are often actually developing theory as they nurse and, in addition, are sometimes basing their practice on existing theories (Benner and Wrubel 1989).

Theory is derived from practice and the most effective care is embedded in expert nursing practice, which is greatly influenced by the context of practical situations. Lauder's position of 'practical wisdom' (1994) brings together theoretical, moral and tacit knowledge, which then provides a union of theory and practice within clinical experience.

Conflicts

Action point

Let's say you want to put some research that you have found into action.

- Are there any constraints that you know of that could prevent you from implementing them?

Nursing is at a crucial stage in its development, and the perception of a theory/practice gap must be of concern to all nurses, whether engaged in clinical practice, education, management or research. Partnership between these important elements of nursing science is vital if we are to provide the very best care possible for our patients.

The move of nurse education into universities has contributed to the perceived widening gap, as has the growing impact of managerialism on UK healthcare. The separation of providers of healthcare (the hospitals and community trusts) and the educators of healthcare must be taken into account, and attempts must be made to reduce the gap. Financial limits and governmental performance targets now heavily influence healthcare. Nurses undertake a great deal of the administration of audits, and budget management is now often devolved to ward level.

All of this would perhaps appear to be in direct conflict with the role of the nurse as intuitive carer, focusing on the patient as an individual person. As long ago as 1972, Briggs commented on the theory/practice gap in nursing, and many other authors have raised numerous complaints that the separation of theory and practice in the classroom setting would only exacerbate this problem. Classroom teaching can never exactly replicate what happens in a range of different clinical areas. However, if theory is explained and examples given from practice to illustrate meanings, this must go some way towards reducing the gap.

Rightly or wrongly, nursing theories are seen to be created by educators and researchers, who tend to live in a different world from those involved in the sometimes harsh reality of clinical practice. There also appears to be a higher level of status attached to nursing theorists than to those who deliver clinical skills, but for many nurses, delivering clinical skills is the most important and rewarding aspect of their work, and indeed is the most valued aspect of the job from the patient's perspective. This situation cannot help when a nurse is unable to utilise theory because it bears no relation to the reality of his or her practice.

Student nurses are encouraged to be independent and enquiring, yet are often considered to have the lowest status within the clinical setting. Although their education and approach to care is based on holistic and humanistic principles, in the organisation-led NHS, the

approach of the mangers sometimes seems to encourage the exact
opposite, that is a task-oriented, functional approach to care. The
potential for philosophical conflict is enormous and often offers
unrealistic goals for students, who then ultimately face disillusion-
ment and disaffection with nursing.

Solutions

The introduction of Project 2000 training was an attempt to reduce
the theory/practice gap, although the higher academic content of
the ensuing curriculum appears to be more theory-focused than ever
before. During the 1980s and 1990s joint appointments such as
lecturer-practitioners were seen as a way forward, ensuring that
teachers were clinically credible and were able to bridge the class-
room-clinical setting divide. Another idea was to increase the time
spent by lecturers as clinical links with community and ward areas,
thereby following the progress and supporting students through
practice experiences.

Reflective practice and research

In recent years, all nurses have been greatly encouraged to use
reflective practice as an educational, personal development tool or
for clinical supervision (Bassett 1999). It has also been suggested as a
method of applying theoretical perspectives to practical experiences
as a way of learning. The role of the student as a catalyst for changing practice based on his or her theoretical knowledge has also been
implicit when educators specifically instruct students to question
practices if they feel they are not based on sound theory. However,
even very experienced nurses are unable to influence change if they
do not have the power and authority in a hierarchical system to do
so.

Increasingly, we hear of the growing professional status of nursing, holistic approaches towards patient care and nurse education,
but arguably this is incongruent with the NHS of today. After 10 or
more years of the market system in health, many healthcare workers
feel alienated and that the caring principles that were the basis of the
NHS have been seriously eroded. Nurse education has quickly
realised that it has a new role as provider in the current marketplace

of education; the educational consortia are the new purchasers, and the services offered by universities need to meet the needs of the hospital and community trusts. This is indeed an opportunity for NHS trusts and other healthcare providers to press for a more practical and evidence-based focus in education provision, and to share equally in that responsibility. Until education and healthcare providers work together and have joint 'ownership' of both pre- and post-registration students the theory/practice gap will continue to exist.

Future initiatives

There are several innovative projects currently in development, one of which is the role of hospital-based clinical demonstrator in Sheffield. This scheme utilises the clinical skills of staff from the ward setting by supporting them in teaching up-to-date, evidence-based skills to students in a clinical skills laboratory (mock ward) setting, alongside experienced teachers. The clinical demonstrators also work in the clinical areas with the same students they have taught in school. This innovation has proved to be an exciting and highly effective innovation for linking school and ward, theory and practice.

Education needs to prepare students to become nurses in the 'real world' as well as giving them the academic preparation needed today. Researchers, educationalists and practitioners seem at times to be working with different imperatives and to have divergent priorities. Is it any wonder that a gap exists? Nursing theories are prescriptive, to be used in the practical application of knowledge in the clinical environment. Practitioners must be aware of and able to choose the most appropriate theoretical principle to use in each situation to achieve the best result for the patient.

Research is often seen as an elitist pastime, irrelevant to everyday clinical practice, yet research without application to the real world is of little use to the nurse caring for patients. It is obvious therefore that researchers and practitioners need to be working in collaboration, or that the two functions need to be invested in the same person. The dissimilar cultures of university (researcher, educator) and clinical (practitioner) setting hold separate values and beliefs, and are believed by many to be different worlds. If the clinician is to utilise research/theory in practice, it is the responsibility of the researcher/educator to ensure there is guidance to enable him or her to do so.

Barriers to research utilisation

A significant barrier to the use of research in practice is the readability of the research findings for those who may wish to apply it. If the academic style and jargon prevent this, then the research is to all intents and purposes lost. Nurses who can write in a nurse-friendly manner are often not encouraged to do so or have little time or inclination, therefore reports are left to academics, for whom it is a requirement to write, in a particularly scholarly and sometimes in incomprehensible, academic style.

It is clear that there is a dilemma for researchers and educators who may have two masters to please. However, the system of nursing should be firmly grounded in practice and academics must never forget this. There is a similar dilemma for students. The disparate cultures of the university and clinical settings clearly exist, but both cultures have to be socialised into. This could be seen as a major contributor to the gap between the development of a nursing research culture and the real practice of nursing. At the moment, the worlds of research and practice are essentially different, but bridging the cultural divide may help to reduce or even close the theory/practice gap. The importance of how research findings are communicated in both content and style cannot be overemphasised – it needs to be clear and accessible to those expected to put it into practice.

Conclusion

In the light of national and regional imperatives for nursing research, a positive research culture must evolve among nurses, encouraged and enabled by researchers, educators and nurse managers. Many trusts now have research strategies for nurses in place in an attempt to do this.

The overall aim of this book is to help redress the balance, giving power to the clinical nurse and enabling the more effective integration of research into the clinical setting. This is essential in today's NHS – the very future of nursing and the first-class care of our patients depends on it.

Action point

- How are you going to deal with the issues surrounding research in practice?
- Are there things you need to do to prepare yourself?
- Chapter 2 expands on these issues, so read on.

References and further reading

Bassett C (1995) Practice development: the sky is the limit. Nursing Standard 9(39): 12-15.

Bassett C (1999) Clinical Supervision a Guide for Implementation. London: NT Books/Emap.

Benner P (1984) From Novice to Expert: excellence and power in clinical nursing. California: Addison-Wesley.

Benner P, Wrubel J (1989) The Primacy of Caring. California: Addison-Wesley.

Briggs A (1972) Department of Health Report on the Committee on Nursing (Briggs Report). London: HMSO.

Carr W (1986) Theories of theory and practice. Journal of Philosophy of Education 20(20): 177-86.

Closs SJ, Cheater FM (1994) Utilisation of nursing research: culture, interest and support. Journal of Advanced Nursing 19: 762-73.

Collins M, Robinson D (1996) Bridging the research-practice gap: the role of the link nurse. Nursing Standard 10(25): 44-6.

Cutcliffe J, Bassett C (1997) Introducing change: the case of research. Journal of Nursing Management 5: 241-7.

Delamothe T (1995) Outcomes into Clinical Practice. London: BMJ Publishing.

Department of Health (1989) Working Paper Ten. London: HMSO.

Department of Health (1991) Research For Health: a research and development strategy for the NHS. London: HMSO.

Department of Health (1992) Health of the Nation. London: HMSO.

Department of Health (1993a) A Vision for the Future: the nursing, midwifery and health visiting contribution to health and health care. London: HMSO.

Department of Health (1993b) Report of the Taskforce on the Strategy for Research in Nursing, Midwifery and Health Visiting. London: HMSO.

Department of Health (1994a) Working in Partnership. London: HMSO.

Department of Health (1994b) Supporting Research and Development in the NHS. A Report for the Minister for Health by a Research and Development Taskforce chaired by Sir Anthony Culyer. London: HMSO.

Ellis R (1992) The practitioner as theorist. In Nichol LH (ed) Perspectives on Nursing Theory, 2nd edn. London: Lippincott.

Greenwood J (1984) Nursing research: a position paper. Journal of Advanced Nursing 9(1): 77-82.

Hunt M (1981) Indicators for nursing practice: the use of research findings. Journal of Advanced Nursing 6(3): 183-94.

Kitson A, Ahmed LA, Harvey G, Seers K, Thompson DR (1996) From research to practice: one organisational model for promoting research based practice. Journal of Advanced Nursing 23: 430-40.

Lauder W (1994) Beyond reflection: practical wisdom and the practical syllogism. Nurse Education Today 14: 91-8.

Lobiondo-Wood E (1986) Nursing Research, Critical Appraisal And Utilisation. New York: Mosby.

National Association of Health Authorities and Trusts (1995) Acting on the Evidence. Birmingham: NAHAT.

NHS Executive (1996) Towards Clinical Effectiveness. London: Department of Health.

Rafferty AM, Allcock N, Lathlean J (1996) The theory/practice 'gap': taking issue with the issue. Journal of Advanced Nursing 23: 685-91.

Trent Regional Health Authority (1993) Every Nurse's Business. Trent Regional Health Authority.

United Kingdom Central Council for Nursing Midwifery and Health Visiting. (1986) Code of Professional Conduct. London: UKCC.

The relevance of research in nursing

TRACEY MOORE

Introduction: the history of nursing research

Florence Nightingale first discussed the importance of applying a research base to nursing practice during the Crimean War. She maintained that practice needed to be up to date and based on the best current research findings available. Unfortunately, for many years afterwards, only minimal reference to nursing research could be found in the nursing literature, and it was not until the 1950s that research reappeared on the nursing agenda.

At this time, several developments within the profession gave impetus to nursing research, including the increased number of nurses with advanced academic training, the development of the *Nursing Research* journal and the availability of funding to support nursing research (Polit and Hungler 1997). In 1972, the Briggs Report urged nurses to keep up to date with research and, as a result, the number of nurses involved in nursing research studies grew significantly. Nurses became key players in discussions relating to theoretical and contextual issues pertinent to their profession. As a consequence, the focus for research studies also changed, and nurses began to examine issues related to the development and improvement of patient care.

The past 20 years have seen growth in the number of nurse researchers, increased involvement of the nurse in research, easier access to research as information technology has developed, increased confidence in conducting research and an overall recognition that research is integral to nursing. Indeed, the status of research in healthcare has helped to place the nurse practitioner at the centre of a healthcare culture that strives for progress and seeks to establish research-based practice.

In essence, the future of nursing research looks, or should look, bright. Yet many argue that, in reality, few nurses actually use research as a basis for practice. They state that many nurses do not know what evidence is available or how to apply it, and that a gap exists between what is known and what is done (Couchman and Dawson 1992).

Take, for example, the findings of the classic study by Hamilton-Smith in 1972. He reported that lengthy preoperative fasting could not be justified for all patients, yet almost 30 years later nurses still complain that this practice persists nationwide, in spite of the evidence.

So why are nurses not using such well-established, readily available research to support their practice?

Traditionally, nurses have been criticised for their resistance to both research and the development of research-based nursing, and their continued support of practices that have no sound research base. Indeed, many practices are founded on custom and tradition alone (Walsh and Ford 1989; Hunt 1997). The reasons nurses fail to use research findings have been discussed frequently in the nursing literature and I am sure you are familiar with those cited: lack of knowledge, disbelief, lack of permission and lack of incentive. But Hunt (1997) argues that these factors alone do not explain fully the limited use of research findings by nurses and that many other barriers to research utilisation need to be addressed if research-based practice is to become widespread.

Perhaps a good starting point would be to examine more clearly what the term 'nursing research' actually means to nurses.

What is nursing research?

It is often suggested that the word 'research' is immediately met with resistance or even 'a frisson of fear' by nurses (Couchman and Dawson 1992). As a result, Robson (1999) suggests replacing the term research with 'enquiry', since he maintains that the two words can be used interchangeably as enquiry can simply be thought of as a way of solving problems. Taking this a step further, enquiry could be likened to a problem-solving model very similar to the one used as part of the nursing process.

Problem-solving model

1 State the problem.
2 Suggest a possible explanation for the problem (formulate a hypothesis).
3 Collect information from observation or experimentation related to the problem.
4 Interpret facts to see if the explanation in step 2 was correct.
5 Make a conclusion about solutions to the problem.

Action point

Think of an example from your clinical practice that you would like to examine. Using the problem-solving model outlined above, move your example through steps 1-5.

Nurses confidently apply the nursing process to their clinical practice daily. Apply the same principles to the research process discussed in Chapter 4, and you will see that the two are in fact very similar. Another way to think about research is to compare it to the work of a detective (Reid 1993). You start with a problem, investigate the problem, build up evidence and then attempt to find a conclusion.

Why do we need research in nursing?

Currently, nursing practice remains a poorly understood phenomenon. Nurses are working within ill-defined boundaries, unclear about what nursing is and what nurses do. Indeed, in the following statement McMahon and Pearson (1991) state that nurses are no different to flight attendants:

> ...the rise in medical knowledge and technology this century has led to the view that 'getting better' or 'staying healthy' is largely dependent on intervention or monitoring by doctors or paramedical therapists and that nurses simply carry out the orders of other professionals and attend to organisational matters. Nurses have become analogous to flight attendants or cabin crew.

So how would you begin to explain what nursing is and what nurses do? Is your role different to a flight attendant or a member of the cabin crew?

You may see from your answer to the above question that the scope of nursing is rather vaguely defined and also constantly changing. If nursing is to be legitimised as a profession then its boundaries need to be defined more clearly. I believe that nurses do have a fairly distinct and unique role in the delivery of healthcare, because unlike many others involved in healthcare delivery, their body of knowledge focuses on the holistic care of the person and their responses to health and illness. Nurses have to examine a person's interaction with the environment in order to help them realise their potential and therefore enable them to find personal growth.

The challenge for nurses is to establish a knowledge base that reflects the depth of their role. They need to provide research information that helps to justify their practice to others and helps to refine, develop and extend the scientific base of knowledge essential to the practice of nursing. For too long practices have been based on custom and tradition. When subjected to research scrutiny, many such practices have fallen foul and have been found to provide no real benefit to patient care as well as being wasteful of time and resources.

For example, Nicky Cullum (1998) told the Directors of Nurse Education annual conference in Cambridge how hundreds of thousands of patients had been dying after myocardial infarctions (MIs) because healthcare professionals had failed to check the available research evidence. It had been known since the 1970s that the use of anti-thrombolytic drugs post-infarction could reduce deaths yet because healthcare professionals failed to look at the evidence systematically, experts did not recognise this specific treatment as being the best. She urged nurses to keep up to date with current research so that they cannot be accused of using ineffective or outdated treatments just because they failed to examine the available evidence.

A common misconception of evidence-based care among nurses is that they have been doing it for years and have been basing their clinical decisions on scientific methods (DiCenso and Cullum 1998). It is estimated that only 20% of medical care is based on statistically sound scientific research and that many interventions are based on intelligent guesswork, clinical hunches and individual clinical skills, which continue despite little evidence to prove their effectiveness (Lewis 1993). Apply this to nursing and the story reads much the same.

Action point

- So how as nurses do we make clinical decisions when we are lacking all the information?
- Make a list of the different strategies you use to make a clinical decision when you are lacking all the information.

The list you come up with may be similar to this one:

- toss a coin
- guess
- use the ethical principle of non-maleficence, i.e. the principle 'to do no harm'
- base it on custom and tradition
- ask colleagues – the problem being that if you ask three colleagues how they would solve the same problem then you are likely to get three different answers
- refer to textbooks (but they may be outdated) (Rourke 1997).

This particular style of decision making is based on the traditional model of medical education, which Rourke (1997) refers to as 'the old model of decision making'.

The assumption is that decision making depends on the facts, principles and conventional practices you develop over the years as a practitioner which, once learnt, will enable you to practise competently for the rest of your professional life. The model maintains that:

- Clinical observation is an effective way of building up knowledge related to patient progress and prognosis.
- New treatments and diagnoses can be evaluated using a combination of traditional medical education and common sense.
- Problems can be answered by asking colleagues or reading textbooks.

The aim of evidence-based practice is to move us away from practice based on ritual and anecdotal experiences to practice that is based on contemporaneous research findings. In line with this, medical education is now moving to a 'new model of decision-making', where the principles state that:

• Clinical experience is still seen as important but observations must now be recorded systematically and without bias.
• Regular reference must be made to original literature.
• The results of studies must be critically examined using the rules of evidence (see Chapter 4) (Rourke 1997).

If nurses are to achieve their professional identity and be truly professionally accountable to patients, then their clinical decisions must also be based on as much scientifically documented evidence as possible. They need to decide what it is that nurses do, so they can enter into a dialogue on what is to be systematically measured and recorded, rather than leaving the measurement up to others, who may be experts at performing research but have little insight into nursing and may not recognise all the important factors. Nurses, whether based in hospital or community settings, are central to nursing research for they are the ones who are in the best position to articulate and evaluate the interventions they use.

Evidence-based practice or evidence-based healthcare, a term more frequently used in the current literature, recognises the pivotal position of the nurse and just like the 'new model of decision-making', it combines nursing expertise with patient preferences, available resources and research evidence. In practising evidence-based healthcare, nurses have to decide whether the evidence is relevant for that particular patient. Their clinical expertise is then balanced against the risks and benefits of alternative treatments for each patient, while also taking into account the patient's own unique circumstances, including co-morbid conditions and preferences. Once these components have been addressed appropriately, the nurse will be in a position to make an effective clinical decision. However, it is important to note that clinical expertise and patient preference may override the other components that constitute evidence-based practice for a given decision. For example, consider the following situation:

Action point

A patient is advised by the practice nurse to give up smoking, following an MI. However, despite the overwhelming evidence that smoking increases the risk of further heart disease and the delivery of an effective health education programme by the nurse, the patient still decides to continue to smoke. That is recognised in the model of evidence-based practice as the patient's preference and his or her decision will override all other components of the model.

All those with a responsibility for patient care are now being urged to ensure that the care they give is evidence-based. Nurses have a professional duty to ensure that the care they deliver is effective. The guidelines for professional practice (UKCC 1996) and the Code of Professional Conduct (UKCC 1992) both state that the registered nurse practitioner is responsible for ensuring that the care given to patients is based on the best-possible up-to-date evidence.

A combination of other forces has also resulted in healthcare professionals being called to demonstrate that the care they provide is both clinically effective and cost-effective. The development of the internal market in healthcare provision and the emergence of NHS trusts and PCGs are just some of the forces that have challenged the healthcare professions (Jack and Oldham 1997).

As the cost of healthcare continues to rise, the need for further cost containment practices is also increasing. As a result, nurses are being asked to document more diligently the social relevancy and the efficacy of their nursing practice to others, such as consumers of nursing care, hospital trust boards and government agencies.

Another reason nurses need to engage in nursing research

The interest in the effectiveness of clinical interventions is also increasing. Clinicians, purchasers, providers and educationalists are all attempting to establish to what extent the care given to patients is based on up-to-date evidence.

Nurses are increasingly focusing their research endeavours on the effectiveness of nursing interventions and activities for various groups of patients, as all those involved in patient care are being urged to ensure that their care is evidence-based (Polit and Hungler 1997).

Many research studies carried out over the past few years have confirmed that patients with the same clinical condition are receiving different types of treatment from practitioners and institutions. For example, a recent audit project undertaken by the Royal College of Nursing (RCN) examined the nursing management of leg ulcers in the community. Their results found inconsistency in practice across the country:

> There is widespread variation in practice, and evidence of unnecessary suffering and costs due to inadequate management of venous leg ulcers in the community.
>
> NHS Centre for Reviews and Dissemination (2000)

In response to their findings, the RCN recommended that a protocol containing evidence-based audit criteria be developed and implemented nationally. The audit results would then be collated nationally to enable comparative data analysis, which would allow individual teams to benchmark their performance against that of others.

Clinical audits and quality assurance mechanisms are tools used to confirm the effectiveness of clinical practice and to highlight any existing deficits in healthcare provision. For example, Waller (1997) explains how nurses in one trust claimed to always give beta-blockers to patients following an MI. On closer examination following a clinical audit trail, it was discovered that only 78% of patients post-MI were receiving the drug.

Clinical effectiveness is about doing the right thing in the right way and at the right time for the right patient (RCN 1996). It measures the extent to which clinical interventions do what they intend to do in relation to maintaining or improving health and achieving the best possible health gain from the available resources. Research plays a major role in achieving these objectives and many examples exist where nurses have been central to furthering the development of clinical practice as a result of research evaluation and application. Examples include such practices as shaving before surgery and the use of cover gowns by nurses when caring for healthy babies in a nursery (DiCenso and Cullum 1998).

With the current changes to the healthcare culture the public sector is now emphasising the importance of open accountability, effectiveness and efficiency. The increasing focus for healthcare professionals therefore is the promotion of better-quality care based on current evidence. Such scrutiny must result in certain aspects of practice being questioned, but if clinical audits show that clinical practice is ineffective, then it enables nurses to take measures to improve their service. Nurses have a responsibility to ensure that the care they give to patients is based on the best possible evidence of effectiveness, and patients have the right to expect this level of care.

Action point

Consider an area of practice that you frequently carry out. Now ask yourself several questions to examine if that practice is evidence-based and clinically effective.

- Are you practising in the right way to achieve the right results for the right patient?
- Are you aware of any up-to-date research studies that have examined this area of practice?
- If so, can you critically appraise the evidence in relation to your practice?
- Has a clinical audit been carried out to find out if the practice is clinically effective?
- Does this practice need changing in any way as a result of your findings?
- Have you shared these changes with your colleagues?

Adapted from *Clinical Effectiveness Resource Pack* (NHS Executive 1997).

The emphasis on evidence-based practice does tend to imply that nurses can access relevant, up-to-date research available in all areas of nursing care, and that they can appraise the evidence and make changes according to the results of their appraisal. But nursing research is still a relatively new phenomenon and as a result, many of the day-to-day activities carried out by nurses have not been subject to formal research study. So what should nurses do when there appears to be no up-to-date evidence on which to base their practice? The NHS Executive (1997) suggests several actions that the nurse practitioner can consider to ensure that he or she is delivering best practice. These include:

- contacting the experts in this field to discuss what they recommend as best practice
- seeking advice from national, regional or local resource centres or individuals
- discussing the practice with colleagues to reach a consensus on what you think best practice should be locally.

Another explanation for the lack of available research for assessing the effectiveness of clinical practice may be the qualitative/quantitative divide in nursing research. Cullum (1998) believes that some nurses have a real antipathy towards quantitative research. Indeed,one of the common misconceptions of nurses concerning evidence-based practice was the overemphasis on randomised controlled trials and systematic reviews (DiCenso and Cullum 1998).

Nurses need to discard their suspicion of scientific, quantitative evidence and instead concentrate on designing imaginative trials which will help them to improve many aspects of nursing, for many questions in nursing lend themselves to quantitative study. Nursing interventions, for example, are best examined using randomised controlled trials and systematic overviews. Consider a study examining the effects of a Mediterranean diet on cardiac mortality and subsequent MI in patients who have had their first MI (de Lorgeril et al. 1998), or one examining the effectiveness of music therapy intervention on relaxation and anxiety for patients receiving ventilatory assistance (Chlan 1998).

Qualitative studies are the best designs for understanding patients' experiences, attitudes and beliefs. Consider a study examining how women experience the presence of their partners at the birth of their babies (Bondas-Salomen 1998), or women's experiences of the menopausal transition (Kittell et al. 1998). Each research design has its strengths and its limitations. The key to success is choosing the right design for answering the question posed.

Action point

Consider an area of practice that you would like study.

• What kind of research design would you use?

• Why would you choose this design?

Accessing information does prove difficult for some nurses where on-site library facilities are lacking or poor. There may also be quite a long time delay between the research being conducted and it being accepted for publication. So by the time research actually reaches the journals it may already be out of date. So how can access be improved?

Recently, several databases have been developed, such as the Cochrane Database, several evidence-based health-related websites and the Health Outcomes Database, which guide the creation, review, maintenance and dissemination of systematic overviews of the effects of healthcare. There are also several newsletters available, such as *A Gathering of Evidence* (newsletter) and The Journal Club on Web, which summarise articles based on rigorous research from major biomedical journals into more concise, meaningful, quick-to-read reports. These newsletters also act as a forum for debate, enabling nurses to discuss best-practice issues with colleagues.

The new 'evidence-based' journals such as *Evidence Based Nursing* provide structured, jargon-free abstracts that are commented upon by clinical experts. These journals aim to disseminate research findings to nurses quickly, to ensure that the research explored remains pertinent and up to date.

Nurses have also suggested that organisational constraints can make it difficult for them to practise evidence-based healthcare (Hunt 1997; Cullum 1998). Institutions such as the Centre for Evidence-Based Nursing and the NHS Centre for Reviews and Dissemination can help nurses to develop evidence-based care within their workplaces. Researchers from the centres work with nurses in practice, other researchers, nurse educators and managers to identify evidence-based practice through primary research and systematic reviews. They also encourage the application of evidence into practice through education and other implementation strategies, such as actively disseminating research findings to the key decision makers in the NHS.

In 1997, the NHS Executive Guidelines on Clinical Effectiveness also urged managers to support nurses in what they described as a key function, their involvement in the design and implementation of clinically and/or cost-effective care.

Evidence-based clinical practice guidelines are another useful tool. They are developed for clinical situations that have already been subject to plenty of rigorous research. The guidelines also demand that variation in practice for patients with the same clinical situation exists. If variation in practice does not exist, then guidelines are not needed. Clinical practice guidelines also have to be multidisciplinary. Nurses and other healthcare professionals interact in order to provide the most effective patient care, so they all need to be involved in the creation of evidence-based guidelines. Indeed, in a multiprofessional healthcare environment it is essential that we look to each discipline for up-to-date evidence on which to base best practice.

So while there are very real reasons for the non-use of research by nurses, there is also evidence that things are improving. The barriers to research utilisation are gradually being dismantled and replaced by a collection of support mechanisms which will help nurses to access, appraise and promote evidence-based practice.

And although it would appear that there is still an uneasy relationship between nurses and research, we have to take strength from the fact that nursing research is a relatively new area. The barriers are gradually being removed and more resources are being made available for providing research advice and support. Nurses are undertaking and completing lots of good research and, while the process may be slow, a research base for nursing practice is gradually developing.

I believe the future for healthcare looks promising as nursing aims to achieve evidence-based practice. This is an exciting development, but the process is clearly complex. There will be problems and disappointments along the way. Establishing evidence-based practice will not be easy, as it demands a change in the present culture. All nurses, irrespective of the sphere in which they work, will be expected to examine their practice in a more systematic way. They will be required to critically appraise research to find best practices and then disseminate and implement these findings to colleagues.

Promoting evidence-based practice will be a challenge, but nurses have a professional duty to ensure that care is delivered effectively. They are responsible for ensuring that patient care is based on the best possible evidence of effectiveness.

Conclusions

- The term 'research' is immediately met with resistance by nurses as it conjures up images of something remote and academic. It is suggested that is replaced with the word 'enquiry', since the two can be used interchangeably. Enquiry is seen as more favourable as it can be likened to a way of simply solving problems.
- Research is needed to define the boundaries of nursing more clearly and so help legitimise the profession.
- There is a need for more research into the way clinical nurses make decisions and the kinds of research needed to help them make these decisions.
- Nurses have a professional duty to ensure that the care they give to patients is based on the best-possible up-to-date evidence.
- Healthcare professionals are being called to demonstrate that their care is both clinically effective and cost-effective. The activities involved in clinical effectiveness include: appraising the evidence; disseminating best practice; changing practice if necessary; and confirming through clinical audit that practice is consistent with best practice.
- Barriers to research utilisation are gradually being dismantled and replaced by a collection of support mechanisms which will help the nurse to access, appraise and promote evidence-based nursing.

References

Bondas-Salomen T (1998) How women experience the presence of their partners at the births of their babies. Qualitative Health Research 8: 784-800.

Chlan L (1998) Effectiveness of a music therapy intervention on relaxation and anxiety for patients receiving ventilatory assistance. Heart and Lung 27: 169-76.

Couchman W, Dawson J (1992) Nursing and Health Care Research. London: Scutari Press.

Cullum N (1998) Evidence-based practice. Nursing Management 5(3): 32-5.

de Lorgeril M, Salen P, Martin JL (1998) Mediterranean dietary pattern in a randomised trial: prolonged survived and possible reduced cancer rate. Archives of Internal Medicine 158: 1181-7.

DiCenso A, Cullum N (1998) Implementing evidence-based nursing: some misconceptions. Evidence-Based Nursing 1(2): 38-40.

Hunt J (1997) Towards evidence based practice. Nursing Managment 4(2): 14-17.

Jack B, Oldham J (1997) Taking steps towards evidence-based practice: a model for implementation. Nurse Researcher 5(1): 65-71.

Kittell LA, Kernoff Mansfield P, Voda AM (1998) Keeping up appearances: the basic social process of the menopausal transition. Qualitative Health Research 8: 618-33.

Lewis B (1993) Diagnostic dilation and curettage in young women. British Medical Journal 306: 225-60.

McMahon R, Pearson A (1991) Nursing as a Therapy. London: Chapman and Hall.

NHS Centre for Reviews and Dissemination (2000) A review of the factors influencing non-recurrence of venous leg ulcers. Database of Abstracts of Reviews of Effectiveness, vol 1. University of York: NHS Centre for Reviews and Dissemination.

NHS Executive (1997) Clinical Effectiveness Resource Pack. Leeds: NHS Executive.

Polit DE, Hungler BP (1997) Essentials of Nursing Research: methods, appraisal and utilization, 4th edn. New York: Lippincott.

Reid N (1993) Health Care Research by Degrees. Oxford: Blackwell.

Robson R (1999) Real World Research. Oxford: Blackwell.

Rourke AO (1997) Seminar 3: an introduction to Evidence-Based Practice. WISDOM Project.

Royal College of Nursing (1996) Clinical Effectiveness: a Royal College of Nursing guide. London: RCN.

UKCC (1992) Code of Professional Conduct. London: UKCC.

UKCC (1996) Guidelines for Professional Practice. London: UKCC.

Waller S (1997) Nurses struggle to use evidence. Nursing Standard 11(28): 8.

Walsh M, Ford P (1989) Nursing Rituals. Oxford: Butterworth-Heinmann.

CHAPTER 3

Commonly used research methods

LORRAINE B ELLIS

Introduction

Clinicians and nurse educationalists are required to produce evidence of research-based practice (Briggs 1972; DoH 1989; Mulhal 1995). This is further endorsed by the Code of Professional Conduct (UKCC 1992), which requires nurses and midwives to provide care that is research-based wherever possible. Research-based care is partly dependent on an appreciation of the methods used to study a given topic. Indeed, the blind application of research findings is at best inadequate and at worst contrary to the provision of quality care. Hence the need for practitioners and educationalists alike to become discerning consumers of research and research methods provides the rationale for this chapter.

Aimed at the consumer, it provides an account of those factors that do and should influence the methodology, and the relationship between the literature review and the research design. The characteristics of qualitative and quantitative research are outlined, together with a broad overview of the most common designs associated with each. The differing ways of researching nursing practice are illustrated using examples, and some of the strengths and limitations of this research is indicated. The value of combining qualitative and quantitative research is considered through specific designs.

Action point.

* What ways of researching have you seen used in your area of nursing practice?

Methodology: choosing an appropriate method

The research design is the outcome of a variety of factors that have helped shape and determine the overall approach and the methods selected. Some of these factors are within the control of the researcher, while others are outside their control. When designing a research project the researcher is faced with a number of choices, some based on factors external to him or her, others based on personal experiences and preferences.

External factors

External factors may include practical issues such as funding and time constraints. The amount of finance granted and the ways in which funds can be used may play a significant part, for example some funding bodies specify a particular research methodology. Similarly, time constraints may be associated with the bid process, where quite often the researcher must develop and submit his or her research proposal within a very short time frame. This can result in little time to develop ideas fully. Often research projects are limited in time by the sponsor who requires the results for a specific event, publication or the launch of a new initiative.

Internal factors

The design may also be influenced by the researcher's personal preferences and past experiences of particular methodologies. These are often the less-obvious reasons for selecting a particular research design, but are no less influential in informing the type of design chosen. In some instances, the researcher may be persuaded to adopt the methodology of the day, there being definite trends in research.

Equally important are those factors that are theoretically rooted and contribute to decisions about the chosen methodology.

Theoretical factors

Morse (1994) suggests, 'The researcher should learn everything possible if he or she is to avoid reinventing the wheel' (p 26). Searching the literature provides the researcher with a sense of what is already known on a given topic.

> **Action point**
> * Can you think of an area of your practice that you would like to explore further?
> * What things would be useful to know that would help you better research the area?

You would be guided in this process by asking yourself:

* What is already known on the subject?
* What am I really trying to find out?

Collectively, internal, external and theoretical factors may be viewed as constraints or opportunities, creating the parameters within which the researcher must design his or her research. Methodological boundaries aside, the important point here is that the critical reader of research should be aware of how these factors may, or indeed should, have influenced the design the researcher finally decided upon.

The relationship between the literature review and the research design

Ascertaining the answers to the previous questions involves the researcher undertaking a critical review of the body of literature on a particular topic and producing a synthesis of the information. The literature review should incorporate all forms of literature, not just those based on empirical research. Searching for and learning all there is to know about the setting, the culture and the study topic serves to help the researcher:

- identify the relevant concepts
- understand the underlying perspectives, beliefs and values of other researchers.

This information is then used to justify the investigation in, for example, the research proposal (Field and Morse 1985).

A critical review of the literature also produces two closely related outcomes: the level of the existing body of knowledge on the topic under investigation, and the key dimensions and indicators of the topic that will inform the development of the data collection methods. This will be covered more fully in Chapter 4. Together these outcomes form the foundation or starting point for the research, creating the theoretical or conceptual framework that guides if not preordains the research design and methodological choices (Ellis and Crookes 1998).

Levels of knowledge and the research design

Importantly, a review of the literature determines the *level* of the existing body of knowledge and therefore provides a rationale or theoretical basis for the research design. DePoy and Gitlin (1994) describe three levels of research design each reflecting the level of the body of knowledge on a particular topic:

- level 1 – exploration
- level 2 – description
- level 3 – prediction.

At the exploratory level there is very little knowledge about the topic under investigation. The researcher will be developing theory and therefore looking to design research that will allow exploration of the topic. Level 1 questions address the lowest and fundamental level of abstractions, such as concepts and constructs. Research questions that build on and refine the results of level 1 knowledge then lead to level 2 or descriptive knowledge. Level 2 research questions are designed to elicit descriptions about the nature, extent or direction of one variable in a population. Once there is a substantive body of knowledge about a phenomenon, either as a single entity or part of a greater context or population, this leads to the development of questions that test knowledge. Research questions aimed at testing knowledge are at the predictive level and reflect research that is designed to determine cause and effect relationships. Thus, each level of knowledge leads to the development of exploratory descriptive or predictive-type designs. Figure 3.1 outlines the three levels, the route of inquiry and the associated features.

The literature review: emerging concepts or indicators

The literature review also produces a series of concepts or constructs about the subject under review. The researcher may then develop or use existing data collection methods that take account of these concepts, building on what is already known. This is perhaps best

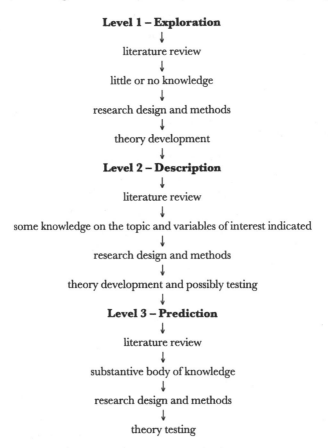

Level 1 – Exploration
↓
literature review
↓
little or no knowledge
↓
research design and methods
↓
theory development
↓
Level 2 – Description
↓
literature review
↓
some knowledge on the topic and variables of interest indicated
↓
research design and methods
↓
theory development and possibly testing
↓
Level 3 – Prediction
↓
literature review
↓
substantive body of knowledge
↓
research design and methods
↓
theory testing

Figure 3.1 Levels of knowledge and the route of enquiry.

illustrated using a specific example. A literature review was carried out as part of a research project funded by the English National Board for Nursing, Midwifery and Health Visiting (Davies et al. 1997b). The project aimed to evaluate the extent to which educational programmes in nursing enable nurses to promote autonomy and independence of older people in their care. This review suggested a range of nursing interventions for promoting patient/client autonomy. These interventions provided the research team with indicators for the concepts of autonomy and independence. These were then operationalized and incorporated into the instruments for data collection, which included a questionnaire and observation tool.

Internal, external and theoretical factors such as those described above, exert an influence on the research design and data-collection methods culminating in an overall approach to the study of a given topic. These approaches are traditionally referred to as qualitative and quantitative.

Overall approaches to research

Action point

- Have you heard about qualitative and quantitative research approaches?
- Write down what you know about these two types of research and try to match up the kinds of clinical problems you know about from your practice setting with the most suitable approach. You may wish to come back to this when you have read the rest of the chapter.

Qualitative and quantitative designs

Whether undertaking research or developing an appreciation of its utility, research is traditionally categorized as quantitative or qualitative. Often these approaches have been viewed as conflicting and competing paradigms, while others would see them as complementary. Indeed, in response to the perceived inadequacies of these approaches, a third paradigm has emerged known as critical social theory or action research (Webb 1989; Wilson-Thomas 1995; Ellis and Crookes 1998). However, caution must be exercised when labelling research, for whether the term quantitative, qualitative or action research is used, these fields are far from a unified set of principles. In real terms, each approach is defined by a series of tensions, contradictions and hesitations that negate absolute categorization. Nonetheless, at the risk of self-contradiction, broadly speaking each of these perspectives reflects a philosophical view of the world or assumptions about how it should be researched.

Perhaps unsurprisingly, given the internal and external factors mentioned previously in this chapter, the characteristics of these world views are a reflection of the values, attitudes, beliefs and expectations associated with each approach. Thus, the research design is a manifestation of a multiplicity of factors that tend to be reduced to the label of quantitative or qualitative. For, whether a seasoned researcher or a student undertaking a research module, when asked how research is traditionally categorized, there is a tendency to think in terms of qualitative and quantitative.

Quantitative and qualitative approaches are associated with particular terms, concepts or notions. Table 3.1 provides a list of the terms normally associated with each approach. This list is a collection of the words compiled by undergraduate and postgraduate students attending research modules.

Interestingly, these lists have remained constant over time, which suggests that the traditional view of research persists, and that the categories are discrete and potentially unrelated.

To help disentangle and make sense of all that research encapsulates, it is perhaps useful to identify the key components or headings associated with any research design. Below is a list of the broad headings that are useful for thinking about research design or strategy:

- The overall research design or strategy.
- Question or hypothesis.
- Population and sample.
- Data collection methods.
- Forms of analysis.
- Data presentation.

These headings provide the essential framework, which helps to signpost the route for considering the appropriateness of each of the

Table 3.1 Terms normally associated with quantitative and qualitative research

Quantitative	Qualitative
Cause and effect	Intuitive
Generalizable	Subjective
Masculine	Interviews
Measurement	Inductive
Statistics	Generating theory
Observable phenomena	Participant observation
Deduction	Soft
Surveys	Heuristic
Systematic	Hermeneutics
Mechanistic	Pluralism
Deterministic	Particular
Causal relationships	Diaries
Hard	Phenomenology
Operational definitions	Interpretive
Hypothesis testing	Naturalistic
Experiment	Grounded theory
Universal laws	Journals
Numerical	Humanistic
Testing theory	Narratives
Positivism	Social sciences
Reductionist	Critical theory
Scientific	Ethnography
Natural sciences	Critical social theory
Randomized controlled trial (RCT)	Feminine

components when reviewing empirical work. This list may also help safeguard the tendency to merely label research quantitative or qualitative without giving considered thought to the respective components.

Qualitative approaches

Qualitative approaches to research, otherwise referred to as naturalistic inquiry, have their origins in the fields of social anthropology and sociology and are associated with the social sciences. Qualitative research is usually adopted when little is known about a given topic and is associated with inductive forms of reasoning in an attempt to generate theory (Ellis and Crookes 1998). Researchers working in this paradigm stress the socially constructed nature of reality, the intimate relationship between the researcher and what is studied, and the situational constraints that shape inquiry (Denzin and Lincoln 1994). This research is usually undertaken in a naturalistic setting where events are normally allowed to take their course unaffected by the research. The context of the research is recognized as an integral part of the phenomenon or topic under investigation and described in considerable detail. This level of detail is important, as it allows the critical reader to consider the appropriateness of the research findings to his or her practice setting. Qualitative research centres on the study of individuals and/or groups of individuals in an attempt to capture their perspective and meanings. Accordingly, all types of sampling are purposeful in qualitative research (Patton 1990), and are otherwise referred to as purposive, judgemental or non-probability sampling. The researcher adopting a qualitative approach aims to make explicit the knowledge, meanings and perspectives known implicitly by those within a particular society (Field and Morse 1985). Thus, qualitative researchers seek answers to questions that stress how experience is created and given meaning.

Several research designs or strategies fall under the heading qualitative research, including grounded theory, phenomenology and ethnography. The following section provides an overview of the characteristics associated with each approach, along with specific examples to illustrate meaning and some of the strengths and limitations. Interestingly, it was not easy to provide examples that fell neatly into the respective approaches, due to the general lack of research that could easily be described as one type of qualitative research or another. Often the researcher used both qualitative and quantitative data collection methods or failed to indicate clearly the research design adopted. Perhaps fortuitously, this process serves to highlight some of the limitations of categorizing research as either qualitative or quantitative.

Grounded theory

Grounded theory was introduced in 1967 by Glaser and Strauss and is described as a form of analysis rather than a distinct qualitative approach (Field and Morse 1985; Morse and Field 1996). Grounded theory has its foundations in the symbolic interactionist perspective (Chenitz and Swanson 1986) that asserts that meaning is socially constructed and changes over time. Participants are selected based on their knowledge of the topic and on the needs of the developing theory, a process known as theoretical sampling (Glaser and Strauss 1967; Glaser 1978; Coyne 1997).

This approach explicitly involves generating theory and doing social research as two parts of the same process. This means that data collection and analysis are undertaken concurrently, each process informing the other. The researcher moves back and forth in the data constantly re-analysing to ensure that all possible explanations have been considered, a process known as constant comparison. The researcher continues to collect data until there is sufficient information to make complete sense of the situation or circumstances. If there are any gaps in understanding the researcher must return to collect further data from the same sample or other informants and this may involve using different data collection methods. This process continues until 'saturation' is reached, where no new themes emerge. Returning to the participants and 'checking out' the meanings attributed by the researcher against those of the participants may verify data analysis. This analytic strategy is otherwise known as 'member checking', and increases the credibility or validity of the research.

Ellis (in preparation), as part of her study, used grounded theory to analyse the transcripts of interviews with nominees ($n = 15$) attending a short course of study and their nominating manager ($n = 19$). *Ellis explored the effects of continuing professional education on nurses using a longitudinal design. She interviewed (audio-taped) the nominees and their managers before the nominee attended a short, focused programme, immediately post-course and six and 12 months post-course. Each transcript was analysed, considered in light of the participant's previous transcripts and used to inform subsequent interviews across the sample, a pattern that was repeated throughout data collection. In this way, the data was constantly compared for similarities and the unique. Verification of findings with participants was not possible due to time constraints and is therefore a limitation of this study.*

Phenomenology

Phenomenological research is the study of everyday experience and an interpretation of the meaning of those experiences as described by the study participants (DePoy and Gitlin 1994). Phenomenology is both a philosophy and a research method that aims to capture the participants' perspective of their 'lived experiences' in the belief that participants' subjective experiences are the only reliable source of information. Information is usually obtained through tape-recorded interviews, which are transcribed verbatim, noting, for example, tone of voice, utterances and general demeanour. Central to phenomenological research is the need to reflect the views of the study participants, hence the tendency to feed back to the participants and 'check out' the respective interpretations. This process of returning to the participants serves to enhance the validity of the research findings, by checking whether the researchers' interpretations of the data are a true reflection of participants' reality.

Bousfield (1997) adopted a phenomenological approach to study clinical nurse specialists' perceptions and experience of their roles. Seven participants were selected from an array of clinical directorates and specialties with differing responsibilities and stages of professional development. Data was collected using interviews (audio-taped) and the interviewees encouraged to express their thoughts and feelings as each part of their role was analysed. The researcher adopted a 'helping status' to facilitate responses and to help the participants to feel comfortable and relaxed (Keenan 1979). The taped interviews were transcribed, analysed and reanalysed and the emerging themes presented. To ensure that the views of the participants were presented as opposed to those of the researcher, Bousfield adopted a system of bracketing. Throughout the research process, Bousfield attempted to 'bracket her own experiential knowledge to capture the empirical reality outside herself' (Swanson-Kauffman and Schonwald 1988). Put differently, the researcher attempted to bracket or suspend and ring-fence their perspective, preventing their beliefs, assumptions and preconceptions about the research topic from impinging on the research. Bracketing is used to help the researcher avoid misinterpreting the phenomenon as the individual is experiencing it, and thereby safeguards the validity of this aspect of the research.

Ethnography

Ethnographic research aims to understand the underlying patterns of behaviour and meaning of a culture (DePoy and Gitlin 1994; Morse and Field 1996). Culture represents a set of explicit and tacit rules, symbols and rituals that guide patterns of behaviour within a group. Complete understanding relies on the researcher having extensive knowledge of the culture. This is often achieved by becoming part of the research setting and observing the environment in which the culture operates. Alternatively, access to the culture may be gained by relying on 'insiders', who willingly engage with the researcher, alert to the culture and the cultural environment. These participants or informants are the researchers 'finger on the pulse of the culture' (DePoy and Gitlin 1994). Once the ethnographer has gained access to the culture, he or she seeks to gain a sense of the cultural context or social scene by observing the environment in which the culture operates. Equipped with an understanding of the cultural context, the researcher then collects data using one or more of the following methods:

- participant observation
- interview
- field notes
- documents and diaries.

Data collection and analysis take place concurrently (Morse and Field 1996) in an attempt to reveal meaning and to generate theory. The ethnographer does not take the data at face value but regards them as inferences from which cultural patterns may be identified and tested (Boyle 1994). Investigator bias may impact on data collection processes and interpretative accounts. To prevent this, the ethnographer sometimes uses reflexivity. The term reflexivity refers to the processes of self-examination and involves the researcher examining how his or her perspective and thinking processes have influenced what is learned and how (DePoy and Gitlin 1994). Reflexive analysis therefore is the extent to which the researcher is conscious of his or her influence on the research process.

Sidenvall et al. (1994) used an ethnographic approach to study the cultural aspects of the effects of the nurses' care actions on the meal situation of hospitalized elderly patients. The research aimed to describe the perceptions of elderly patients and staff towards patient meal times and collective dining, and explore the congruence between these perceptions. The sample consisted of 18 patients and 21 nurses taken from rehabilitation and long-term care wards. Sample selection criteria included patients who were mentally orientated. Patients' admission diagnoses included Parkinson's disease, cerebral vascular accident, fractured hip and spondylarthrosis. Data collection methods included a combination of participant observation, interviews and nursing records documentation on patients' eating and eating prescriptions. One of the limitations of Sidenvall's research was its limited application beyond the culture under investigation – the work was carried out in Sweden, where the cultural values and norms underpinning the care of the elderly may be very different from other cultures. Accordingly, the 'cultural gap' may be such that the research findings have limited, if any, application in the UK.

The appropriateness of the role of the researcher observing patients during meal times is also questionable. Meal times are usually private and not normally associated with spectators. Moreover, interview extracts suggest that in trying to feed themselves, some of these patients were struggling to maintain their sense of dignity and self-respect. Ethnographic research stresses the importance of the relationship between the researcher and the participants, the researcher becoming part of the research setting. Clearly, the study of the meal situation in elderly care did not comply fully with the philosophy of a true ethnographic approach. Nonetheless, Sidenvall (1994) and her colleagues built on a very limited body of knowledge on the meal-time experience of the elderly and therefore contributed to theory development on this issue.

Quantitative approaches

Quantitative research is founded on positivism, a philosophy that is usually associated with the scientific method (Bryman 1988). It has its roots in the natural sciences and is concerned with measurement. A characteristic of the scientific method is its emphasis on systematic and controlled procedures for acquiring dependable, empirical information (Polit and Hungler 1993). The relationship between the researcher and the research subjects is often one of detachment. This is reflected in the terms sometimes used to describe those who are a source of data, the quantitative researcher referring to them as subjects or respondents as opposed to participants. Broadly speaking, quantitative research tends to be adopted when there is a substantive body of knowledge on a given topic, and the variables of interest are subject to control and manipulation. Quantitative research is associated with deductive patterns of reasoning and theory testing (see for example Ellis and Crookes 1998), and is designed to describe and test the effects of one or more variables on another determining a cause and effect relationship.

There are a range of quantitative research designs, including, for example, experimental, quasi-experimental, correlational and survey. Despite their number and diversity, the tendency is to associate quantitative research with the experiment and the survey. The characteristics of each along with examples are presented below.

Experiments

The experiment is often seen as the archetype of quantitative research and the terms are used interchangeably. Experimental research is also referred to as:

- the randomized control trial (RCT)
- clinical trials
- pre- and post-test control group design
- the scientific method.

Whether described as an RCT or clinical trials, the experiment is characterized by randomization, control and manipulation (Campbell and Stanley 1963; Polit and Hungler 1991). Randomization or random sampling is a mechanism for control in quantitative research, which usually provides a sample that is representative of a population. A representative sample is acquired since each member of the population is selected independently and has an equal chance or probability of being included in the study. Thus, experimental research uses probability sampling.

Control involves the researcher imposing rules to decrease the possibility of error and therefore increase the likelihood or probability that the findings are an accurate reflection of reality. The degree of control possible will vary according to the setting. In some settings, the control will be partial and in others highly controlled. The RCT is sometimes referred to as 'hard' science, and is usually associated with research undertaken in a laboratory setting (Burns and Grove 1993). Here the researcher has considerable control over the environment and conditions. Highly controlled settings reduce the influence of extraneous variables, which enables the researcher to examine accurately the effect of the independent variable on the dependent variable. Put differently, through control, the researcher can reduce the effects of extraneous and confounding variables on the research variables. Control and manipulation are characteristics of the RCT that are closely linked. The researcher controls and modifies the environment introducing the independent variable or intervention then measures the effect.

Exercising control over research undertaken in a laboratory using, for example, chemicals or animals, is relatively easy and straightforward. However, the converse is true in the study of people who are inherently different, and the issue of control over human beings raising ethical and moral questions. Furthermore, producing the controlled research environment that the RCT demands is extremely difficult to achieve in a reality that is often characterized by disorder and far more 'messy' (see Ellis et al. 2000). Some of the difficulties of applying an experiment in a social setting are illustrated in a study by Davies et al. (1997a). They designed an RCT to evaluate the effects of a short, focused programme (ENB 941 Nursing Elderly People) of continuing professional education on nursing practice. The research was designed to test the following hypothesis:

> Nurses who have undertaken the ENB 941 Course (Nursing Elderly People) are more likely to promote autonomy and independence in their practice with older people than nurses who have not undertaken the programme.

Course members were to be allocated at random to either an experimental or a control group from a list of potential nominees identified by nurse managers. The experimental group would then undertake the next available programme and the control group would be offered places on the following programme. Table 3.2 summarizes the proposed research design and data collection methods.

Both groups would complete structured questionnaires before and after the experimental group undertook the ENB 941 programme. A subsample of both groups would also be observed in practice before and after the introduction of the independent variable (ENB 941) to the experimental group. Participants would be observed using a rating scale based on the work of Gilloran et al. (1994). Pre- and post-course questionnaires and observations would

Table 3.2 Proposed research design

	Pre-test* Questionnaire $n > 60$	Intervention	Post-test* Questionnaire $n > 60$
Experimental group	Structured non-participant observation $n > 30$ (subsample)	ENB 941	Structured non-participant observation $n > 30$ (subsample)
			Semi-structured interviews with participants, course teacher, nurse manager
	Questionnaire $n > 60$		Questionnaire $n > 60$
Control group	Structured non-participant $n > 30$ observation		Structured non-participant $n > 30$ observation

be complemented by brief semi-structured interviews with course members and their nurse manager in the practice setting to explore their perceptions of the impact of the course on practice.

Adhering to the principles of the RCT was problematic in the context of this research and for the following reasons.

Randomization

Setting up the RCT was dependent on recruiting a sufficiently large sample that was to be generated from several centres offering the ENB 941 and within the time frame of the study. However:

- not all centres offered the ENB 941
- there was no waiting list of course applicants
- several applicants had been waiting to attend the 941 for some time and were reluctant to the possibility that their application may be deferred to the following course
- there was a decline in the number of places offered.

Control and manipulation

Generating a sufficiently large sample meant recruiting from several centres offering the course. While all the 941 programmes were validated by the ENB, the programmes differed considerably, both in the number of study days, duration, philosophy, content and the number of credits. This meant that the sample would not receive the same treatment or independent variable. Clearly the 941 was not subject to the manipulation and control that the RCT demands, and the lack of a standard intervention would therefore compromise and potentially invalidate the results.

Together, these factors and others meant that Davies et al. (1997) resolved to adopt a quasi-experiment to evaluate the effects of the ENB 941. Quasi-experimental designs look much like an experiment but lack either the randomization or control-group feature that characterizes true experiments. Research lacking in these characteristics is said to weaken the researcher's ability to make causal inferences (Polit and Hungler 1993).

Surveys

Definitions of survey research are many and varied (Moser and Kalton 1993), with some writers using the negative definition of 'non-experimental' (LoBiondo-Wood and Haber 1994; Polit and Hungler 1993; DePoy and Gitlin 1994). Survey research is perhaps best defined in terms of its purpose, this being primarily to measure the characteristics of a population, for example age, occupation, number of dependants, etc. The earliest surveys were censuses involving all members of the population – one of the first was the Doomsday survey. Possibly the most common types of survey today include General Household Surveys, Gallup polls and market research.

There are two broad types of survey design, those that describe the characteristics of the population and those that suggest possible relationships among those characteristics. Surveys have a capacity for generating quantifiable data on large numbers of people and therefore are typically associated with large samples. Having said this, survey research nearly always uses a proportion of the population and seeks to represent the characteristics of the population so that findings can be generalized (Thomson 1998).

Survey design can be classed as one-shot, time-series or repeated-contact (Campbell and Stanley 1963). One-shot design is where the researcher collects all the information needed from the sample of a population at a given point in time. Time-series design aims to

examine changes in the population pertaining to a given phenomenon over time, and the data are collected from different subjects of
the population at preset time intervals. Similar to the longitudinal
design, repeated contact involves the researcher collecting information from the same sample on two or more occasions. This approach
is concerned with change over a period of time and may, for example, centre on changes in attitudes, perceptions and behaviour.
However, unlike experimental research, it is not possible to assert a
true cause-and-effect relationship. Survey data-collection methods
include self-completion questionnaires and interviews.

Mackintosh and Bowles (1997) adopted a time-series design to
measure and evaluate the impact of a nurse-led inpatient acute pain
control service on postoperative pain control. A baseline survey was
carried out before the service was introduced in 1992 using a
random sample of 100 patients. The survey was then replicated in
1995, again using a random sample of 106 patients taken from the
same ward areas undergoing the same range of procedures as in the
first study. Data-collection methods included a structured interview
and questionnaire covering three areas: pre-operative information
given, actual pain reported and analgesia given. The survey
approach used in this study could not control the many variables that
may have affected patients' perception of pain. However, this type of
research did provide an opportunity to assess a large random sample
of the inpatient population at two points in time before and after the
introduction of change.

The strengths and limitations of the survey method are further
outlined by DePoy and Gitlin (1994, p 117).

Why we need both approaches: beyond the quantitative and qualitative debate

Philosophical and ideological debates on the merits, appropriateness
and application of qualitative and quantitative nursing research
abound in nursing and related literature (Bryman 1984, 1988;
Duffy 1985; Corner 1991; Carr 1994; Clarke 1995; Ellis 1996).
Much of the debate centres on the adherence to scientific principles
and the relationship between research and the development of a
professional body of knowledge. The importance of these issues is
not disputed here. Indeed, awareness of the broad political context

in which the research may be located is crucial to the development of a critical reader. However, there is a need to go beyond the quantitative and qualitative debate (Corner 1991) and to separate out the philosophical or epistemological issues (theory of knowledge) from the technical (Bryman 1984). By technical, Bryman (1984) is referring to the research methods that are used to answer a particular research question. Clearly, in this context the emphasis is on designing research that is fit for the purpose, based on an understanding of the strengths and limitations of quantitative and qualitative research.

A 'fitness-for-purpose' research design may result in the use of an integrated or eclectic approach where methodologies are used to advantage, rather than played against each other.

Integrated design strategies

Earlier in this chapter it was suggested that investigators design their research based on two questions: 'What is already known on the subject?' and 'What am I trying to find out?' Answering these questions produces research that is the outcome of theoretical considerations that lead to the generation or testing of theory. Unencumbered by external and internal factors, the researcher draws on the range of quantitative and qualitative methods to design his or her study, producing an integrated approach. Triangulation is the combination of designs and methods in the study of the same phenomenon (Denzin 1978), so that the advantages of each complement the other, while the inadequacies of individual approaches are offset (Corner 1991). Action research and case study are approaches incorporating features of quantitative and qualitative designs.

Action research

This approach goes by many names, including critical theory or critical social theory. Action research is a relatively new type of design, often referred to as the third research paradigm, and its primary aim is to improve practical situations (Webb 1990; Elliot 1991). Critical theory is distinct from other paradigms in two respects: the purpose of the research per se and the role of the researcher in achieving that purpose (Ellis and Crookes 1998). Action research, as its name suggests, is about introducing change through the empowerment of the research participants. The researcher is an active participant in the research, which involves the participants acting as collective change agents throughout the research process. It is this collectivity which reflects the philosophical assumptions underpinning action research. For, in an attempt to reconcile the customary power imbalance between the researcher and the researched (Ellis and Crookes 1998), the investigator seeks to foster a sense of ownership for the research findings and encourages their application in practice.

Compared with other types of research there are few examples of critical social theory. Using action research, Webb (1989) sought to introduce a change in the patterns of delivery of care from task-orientated to patient-orientated. She provided a detailed account of her role as participant observer and the process of familiarizing herself with the practice environment. She also used questionnaires and interviews to elucidate the perceived priority areas of care. The success of action research is partly dependent on becoming integrated or accepted as a member of the setting, in this instance the ward team. However, herein lie some of the inherent difficulties and limitations of action research. Integration, whilst crucial to the success of action research, raises questions of validity. Validity in action research is established by the processes of self-validity, participant validity and peer validity (Titchen 1995), although these are very time-consuming and therefore a potential disadvantage of this paradigm. This is perhaps best illustrated by Webb (1989), whose study lasted over two years.

Case study

Case studies are in-depth investigations of an individual, group, institution or other social unit (Polit and Hungler 1993). The case study was particularly evident in early nursing research and was used to study nursing interventions (Burns and Grove 1993). The emphasis is on providing a thorough and detailed account of the 'case', the researcher intensively exploring a single unit of study or a very small number of participants (Burns and Grove 1993). The research design may consist of multiple cases that involve a comprehensive examination and comparison of the smaller units that make up each case. Yin (1984) asserts that case study research is particularly appropriate for evaluation purposes since it requires the analysis of contemporary phenomena within their 'real-life' contexts. Accordingly, the case study approach to evaluation takes account of the various perspectives and processes resulting from the intervention. Case study research is amenable to most data-collection methods, including questionnaires and interviews, observation, rating devices, personal documents such as diaries or letters, statistical records and so forth.

A good example of case study design is provided by Billings (1996), who was concerned with developing a community profile (single case study or unit of analysis) that would contain all the necessary information for a healthcare needs assessment by community practitioners. Billings drew on a variety of sources to produce the community profile. Data-collection methods included documentary analysis of epidemiological and antenatal statistical data, health visitor case and field notes, telephone interviews and group interviews with the community school and psychiatric nurses. Billings also provide a useful critique of the case study design through an account of the processes involved in developing the case or community profile.

Action point

Research and its terminology can be daunting. However, if you do not panic when confronted with an unknown word or term and instead look it up and do some further reading, you will develop a clearer understanding of research.

Summary

This chapter provides a broad overview of the most commonly used research designs and associated methods. It considers those factors that influence the choice of design and the tendency to locate research either in a qualitative or quantitative paradigm. It is important for the critical reader of research to identify the research design rather than categorize research according to paradigm only. This will help to discern the match between the research question or hypothesis and the design and route of inquiry.

The chapter also outlines integrated strategies demonstrating the value of combining methods and, through examples, illustrates the strengths and limitations of qualitative, quantitative and integrated research. It is hoped that in completing this chapter the reader, as a key link in the theory (research) practice chain, will use its contents to help determine the value and therefore utility of research and research findings.

References

Billings JR (1996) Investigating the process of community profile compilation. Nursing Times Research 1(4): 270-83.

Bousfield C (1997) A phenomenological investigation into the role of the clinical nurse specialist. Journal of Advanced Nursing 25: 245-56.

Boyle JS (1994) Styles of ethnography. In Morse JM (ed) Critical Issues in Qualitative Research Methods, pp 159-85. Thousand Oaks, CA: Sage.

Briggs, A (1972) Report of the Committee on Nursing. Cmnd 5115. London: HMSO.

Bryman A (1984) The debate about quantitative and qualitative research: a question of method or epistemology? British Journal of Sociology 35(1): 75-92.

Bryman A (1988) Quantity and Quality in Social Research. Contemporary Social Research 18. London: Routledge.

Burns N, Grove SK (1993) The Practice of Nursing Research: conduct, critique and utilisation, 2nd edn. London: Saunders.

Carr LT (1994) The strengths and weaknesses of quantitative and qualitative research: what method for nursing. Journal of Advanced Nursing 20: 716-21.

Campbell DT, Stanley JC (1963) Experimental and Quasi-experimental Designs for Research. Chicago: Rand McNally.

Chenitz WC, Swanson JM (1986) Qualitative research using grounded theory. In Chenitz WC, Swanson JM (eds) From Practice to Grounded Theory. Menlo Park, CA: Addison Wesley.

Clarke L (1995) Nursing research: science, visions and telling stories. Journal of Advanced Nursing 21: 584-93.

Corner J (1991) In search of more complete answers to research questions. Quantitative versus qualitative research methods: is there a way forward? Journal of Advanced Nursing 16: 718-27.

Coyne IT (1997) Sampling in qualitative research. Purposeful and theoretical sampling; merging or clear boundaries? Journal of Advanced Nursing 26: 623-30.

Davies S, Ellis L, Laker S (1997a) Evaluation of pre- and post-registration preparation for the care of older people. Report for the English National Board (ENB) for Nursing Midwifery and Health Visiting.

Davies S, Ellis L, Laker S (1997b) Promoting autonomy and independence for older people within nursing practice: a literature review. Journal of Advanced Nursing Studies 26: 408-17.

Denzin NK (1978) The Research Act: a theoretical introduction to sociological methods. New York: McGraw Hill.

Denzin NK, Lincoln YS (1994) Handbook of Qualitative Research. London: Sage.

Department of Health. (1989) A Strategy for Nursing: report of the steering committee. London: HMSO.

DePoy E, Gitlin LN (1994) Introduction to Research: multiple strategies for health and human services. St Louis, MO: Mosby.

Duffy ME (1985) Designing nursing research: the qualitative-quantitative debate. Journal of Advanced Nursing 10: 225-32.

Elliot J (1991) Action Research for Educational Change. Milton Keynes: Open University Press.

Ellis LB (1996) Evaluating the effects of continuing nurse education on practice: researching for impact. Nursing Times Research 1(4): 296-305.

Ellis LB (in preparation) Continuing professional education for nurses: an illuminative case study. PhD thesis, University of Sheffield.

Ellis LB, Crookes PA (1998) Philosophical and theoretical underpinnings of research. In Crookes PA and Davies S (eds) Research into Practice: essential skills for reading and applying research in nursing and health care, vol 4, pp 85-115. London: Ballière Tindall.

Ellis LB, Davies S, Laker S (2000) Attempting to set up a randomised controlled trial. Nursing Standard 14(21): 32-6.

Field PA, Morse JM (1985) Nursing Research: the application of qualitative approaches. London: Croom Helm.

Gilloran A, McGlew T, McKee K, Robertson A, Wight D (1994) Measuring the quality of care in psychogeriatric wards. Journal of Advanced Nursing 18: 269-75.

Glaser B (1978) Theoretical Sensitivity: advances in the methodology of grounded theory. Mill Valley, CA: The Sociology Press.

Glaser B, Strauss A (1967) The Discovery of Grounded Theory. Chicago: Aldine.

Keenan A (1979) Effects of non verbal behaviour on interviews of candidates' performance. Journal of Occupational Psychology 49: 171-6.

LoBiondo-Wood G, Haber J (1994) Non experimental designs. In LoBiondo-Wood G, Haber J (eds) Nursing Research, Methods, Critical Appraisal and Utilisation, 3rd edn. St Louis, MO: Mosby.

Mackintosh C, Bowles S (1997) Evaluation of a nurse-led acute pain service. Can clinical nurse specialists make a difference? Journal of Advanced Nursing 25: 30-7.

Morse D, Field JM (1996) What is a method? Qualitative Health Research 6(3): 467-8.

Morse J (1994) Emerging from the data: the cognitive processes of analysis in qualitative inquiry. In Morse J (ed) Critical Research Issues in Qualitative Research Methods. Thousand Oaks, CA: Sage.

Moser CA, Kalton G (1993) Survey Methods in Social Investigation. New York: Basic Books.

Mulhal A (1995) Nursing research: what difference does it make? Journal of Advanced Nursing 21: 576-83.

Patton MQ (1990) Qualitative Evaluation and Research Methods, 2nd edn. Newbury Park, CA: Sage.

Polit DF, Hungler BP (1993) Essentials of Nursing Research: methods, appraisal, and utilisation, 3rd edn. London: Lippincott.

Polit DF, Hungler BP (1991) Nursing Research: principles and methods, 4th edn. PA: Lippincott.

Sidenvall B, Fjellstrom C, Christina A (1994) The meal situation in geriatric care – intentions and experiences. Journal of Advanced Nursing 20: 613-21.

Swanson-Kauffman P, Schonwald E (1988) Phenomenology. Paths in Knowledge – innovative research methods. New York: National League for Nursing.

Thomson A (1998) Recognising research processes in research-based literature. In Crookes PA, Davies S (eds) Research into Practice: essential skills for reading and applying research in nursing and health care, vol 5, pp 116-38. London: Ballière Tindall.

Titchen A (1995) Issues of validity in action research. Nurse Researcher 4(5): 327-34.

United Kingdom Central Council for Nurses Midwives and Health Visitors (1992) Code of Professional Conduct. London: UKCC

Webb C (1989) Action research: philosophy, methods and personal experiences. Journal of Advanced Nursing 14: 403-10.

Webb C (1990) Partners in Research. Nursing Times 86(32): 40-4.

Wilson-Thomas L (1995) Applying critical social theory in nursing education to bridge the gap between theory, research and practice. Journal of Advanced Nursing 21: 568-75.

Yin R (1984) Case Study Research: design and methods. London: Sage.

Further reading

Crookes PA, Davies S (1998) Research into Practice: essential skills for reading and applying research in nursing and health care. London: Ballière Tindall.

This book provides a detailed and comprehensive account of the processes outlined in this chapter. In particular, the readers' attention is drawn to Chapters 4 through to 8, as each discusses components of the research process pertinent to the debate on the use of quantitative and qualitative methodology. It also provides details on those designs and methods beyond the scope of this chapter but no less important to the critical reader of research.

Woods NF (1988) Analysing existing knowledge. In Woods NF, Catanzaro M (eds) Nursing Research: theory and practice, pp 46-65. St Louis, MO: Mosby.

CHAPTER FOUR

Reading and understanding research reports

MARK LIMB

Introduction

Current changes in healthcare and nurse education have resulted in an ever-increasing number of research reports being published in both books and healthcare journals. The changes have also led to a different style of education for nurses. Within the academic system of education, students are encouraged not to accept research at face value, but to examine it critically before believing that it can be of use in practice. This means that nurses have to develop different skills to enable them to undertake this important function. Nurses must not assume that all research is good and that it can be used in their own sphere of practice without first checking its rigour and accuracy.

Action point

- Have you recently read any research reports?
- Did you find them easy or difficult to understand?
- It may be useful at this point to seek out an article or two from the journals – make them applicable to your practice area.
- When you have read them make notes about their strengths and weaknesses.
- Now read this chapter, then reread the research and see if it is clearer.

This chapter aims to provide the nurse with some insight into how a research report should be read. First, it may be useful to assess why some nurses avoid reading published research. Lewis and Barnes (1997) provide us with a useful list of reasons for consideration:

* fear of statistical content
* inadequate knowledge of process
* lack of understanding of jargon
* some concepts may be difficult to master.

What do these mean in practical terms and how can they be addressed?

Some people do not like statistics because they can be confusing. However, deciding whether or not a piece of research is good has to be based on objective evidence and not preference or feelings. In addition, it is not absolutely necessary to know all statistical tests and rules to be able to critique quantitative research. Some important issues for the nurse new to critiquing research will be addressed as a starting point in this chapter.

Polit and Hungler (1997) and Hibbert and Crookes (1998) both point out that to critique research there has to be an understanding of the methods used. However, this may not help nurses who feel they have inadequate knowledge of the research process. The discussion in this chapter attempts to move through the process in a methodical manner to try to help put things into the longitudinal perspective that the researcher should have followed.

Unfortunately many research processes will have associated terminology that may seem like jargon at first. It may be unavoidable in some instances, but where possible within this chapter, explanations will be given to aid your understanding.

Some of the ideas and processes in research may be difficult to master. For example, what is the theoretical framework and why is it important? Again such concepts will be explained and reasons for their importance given.

Why critique?

The next important thing to consider is why should we critique research? An important issue here is that the nurse needs to be able to appropriately apply knowledge to practice. Santy and Kneale (1998) tie this into clinical effectiveness, supporting the view of Kneale and Knight (1997) that this involves the application of research knowledge to practice. However, they further warn that skills to review, evaluate and interpret the literature are important to enable the nurse to do this effectively. Research findings should not be blindly accepted.

In support of the above views on clinical effectiveness, Polgar and Thomas (1995) point out that it is important to identify the strengths and weaknesses of a publication to ensure that patients receive treatments and assessment based on the best available evidence. It would be useful for you to consider what you would do if you had two pieces of research on one aspect of practice each with different outcomes. Which one would you use, and why?

If we are to apply research to practice, before we do so we should note, as Lewis and Barnes (1997) point out, that research is conducted in an imperfect world. In view of this, bias may be introduced, mistakes can be made and findings not identified or fairly attributed. Therefore it is important to critique research to appreciate its true worth.

What is a critique?

Next we have to ask ourselves what a critique is. There are many associated terms in the literature such as critical analysis, review, evaluation and appraisal. These can be confusing to the nurse not familiar with some concepts and may need further clarification.

Most nurses will be familiar with the term critical analysis, which Hibbert and Crookes (1998) define as breaking down and examining in detail something both in terms of its parts and how they fit together. Any student undertaking an academic programme of study will undertake this sort of process. Hibbert and Crookes identify the difference between this and critique. They feel that critique requires advanced knowledge of research ethics and methodologies.

Reviewing can also be defined in a different manner. Davies (1998) discusses both literature and systematic reviews. Again most students undertaking academic programmes of study will be familiar with the literature review, whereby the content of all types of literature on a given topic is considered. Systematic reviews are different as this involves identifying the research on a given topic using strict inclusion and exclusion criteria and synthesizing the findings. See Davies (1998) for a more in-depth discussion of these issues.

Critical evaluation is defined by Polgar and Thomas (1995) as identifying the strengths and weaknesses of a piece of research. Lewis and Barnes (1997) feel evaluation is a broader term than critique, although it conveys the same meaning. They feel critiquing entails having an objective and balanced approach when evaluating a piece of research by highlighting its merits and limitations. It is slightly confusing though, as they feel evaluation is a broader term but use it in the definition.

Importantly, Polit and Hungler (1997) point out what critique is not. They state that it is not a review or summary of an individual piece of work. It is not sufficient for the reader to list how the research was undertaken and what the findings were. What is more important is to ascertain whether or not the findings are believable.

After considering the above, it seems that critiquing research is a process of examining the parts of a single report, giving consideration to the individual parts of the report with reference to the theory on how research should be undertaken. Based on this, the reader should give consideration to the strengths and weaknesses inherent within the report that may influence its believability/accuracy.

The parts for consideration

Many books on research contain sections on critiquing published papers, each with different views on what should be considered and which parts may be more important. Some authors further conceptualize the parts into broader headings. For example, Polit and Hungler (1997) talk about the substantive and theoretical, the methodological, the ethical, the interpretative, and the presentation and stylistic dimensions. This can further confuse the nurse new to the process of critiquing research.

The following attempts to draw together the different aspects of research, and is presented in the linear manner in which the research may have been undertaken or presented. It places no emphasis on which aspect is most important, as to omit any aspect would cause problems in understanding. Therefore all aspects of research have to be seen as equally important.

The author(s)

It is always useful to start by looking at who has written the article for publication. Consider the following:

- Who are the author(s) and what are their job title(s)?
- What are their qualifications?

One would assume that if a person holds a respected job within a respected institution and holds qualifications that indicate he or she is well-trained in research processes, it follows that the published research is credible. However, one needs to approach this aspect with caution and consider whether or not the research:

- has been undertaken rigorously and not rushed to produce quick results for personal gain
- has been published because the person is held in high esteem by the academic community and publishers want to have work by such authors in their books/journals, and not because the research process was rigorously undertaken.

The title

What does this convey? Does it strike you as interesting and relevant to your area of nursing practice? Too much jargon may put potential readers off, especially if it is written in such a way that it detracts from, rather than facilitates, the rapid grasp of the essence of the paper. The title should convey a general idea of the research question and methods used.

The abstract

If the title has attracted the attention of the reader the next thing that needs consideration is the abstract. This can be considered as an expansion of the general themes of the title and a condensation of the main report. Effectively, what the writer should be doing is enticing the potential reader to read on. This section should therefore contain a précis of the research question, the methods used and the findings, and it should be written clearly and succinctly.

The introduction and background to the study

At this point it is important to give consideration to why the research was undertaken in the first place. The author should have given some idea of what problem in practice led to the development of the study. It is not acceptable that ideas just come out of somebody's head. In order for it to be relevant and important, the idea for the research must come from some event or problem in clinical practice. The author should have clearly identified this in the report so that the reader is able to:

- establish that the research was required in the first place, and that the cost and effort were justified because it could potentially lead to more effective practice, and was not merely a notion that somebody grasped for the sake of it
- establish whether or not the problem experienced is similar to his or her own, and assess whether or not the study findings will be suitable for generalisation into his or her own particular area.

So this section should contain sufficient information for the reader to be able to grasp the scope and significance of the problem. The problem identified should be specific and tangible rather than general, as this would indicate that the researcher had a clear focus for the study.

Importantly, the reader should also consider whether or not the problem is related to nursing or should really have been undertaken by some other discipline more suited to research into the topic. The reader should note any inadequacies in this section as it could signal that the research was not well-conceived and was, therefore, poorly planned.

The literature review

Given that the problem has been identified and introduced, the author should then show evidence that he or she has undertaken comprehensive reading around the problem. All literature relating to the problem should have been systematically critiqued; this should include review articles and opinion articles, but more importantly the research already undertaken around the problem area. Any research previously undertaken should have been considered in light of research theory to determine its quality and assess whether or not a different approach could have been undertaken for the study. This allows the author to present the reader with a balanced view of the ideas and findings of other authors. Important things to consider here are:

- Have any important works from the literature been omitted?
- What is the attitude to any unfavourable evidence?
- Have general problems in the literature been discussed specifically in relation to the problem under study?
- Given what is known already, is the research undertaken another step to expand the knowledge base of nursing?

Effectively what the researcher should be demonstrating through the literature review is that a problem has been identified for which the current literature either did, or did not, provide a satisfactory solution. If a solution was not available, further research may provide an answer. If a solution was available, the researcher may have wanted to replicate a study. While this may be seen as replication of knowledge and therefore not developing what is currently known, it can increase the generalizability of findings if they are similar to those already reported.

The theoretical framework

Having identified a problem and reviewed the associated literature, the researcher should then have developed a theoretical framework to use as a guide for the study. This should include:

- A description of the concepts under study. This is important, as the researcher should be perfectly clear on exactly what is to be investigated. Operational definitions should have been provided for all variables measured or manipulated. For example, if the study was to examine the relationship between body image and self-esteem, then the researcher must have clearly identified the conceptual definitions of body image and self-esteem. In addition, there may, for example, have been a need to clarify how the researcher was differentiating between lowered self-esteem and depression (which are arguably theoretically different concepts). If the literature review is adequate then this will be obvious. The definition of the concepts will drive the type of measurement tool used, therefore one cannot overemphasize the importance of the soundness of the concepts. If the measurement tool is inappropriate it will affect the validity of the study (does the study measure what it sets out to measure?).

- Any ideas about proposed relationships between the concepts or the effects of one upon another. These may have come from issues arising in practice or they may be drawn from or identified in the literature. These proposed relationships/effects should have been used as hypotheses for the study. The researcher should have stated these clearly as formalized predictions of the relationships or effects of the variables under study. If he or she has not, then the evidence obtained from the study cannot be used effectively for conceptual advances.

Ethical issues

Much of the research undertaken in hospitals and the community is carried out using patients, who are a vulnerable group, particularly if they are ill. The rights of human subjects have to be respected and the following points should have been considered. There should be evidence that:

- informed consent has been obtained
- the subjects were free from harm and coercion
- steps have been taken to ensure the protection of the subjects' privacy, anonymity and confidentiality.

Any sponsorship from outside bodies should have been listed, as this may affect the credibility of the study. An example of this may be when a drug company sponsors research into one of its own products; there may be some pressure on the researcher to try to produce positive results as this may affect their profit levels.

In particular, you should consider the scientific merit of the study compared with the wellbeing of the subject. From reading the research report, which of these two do you feel is given priority?

The sample and setting

First, the paper should provide a description of the population from which the sample has been drawn, as this provisionally enables the reader to decide if it is a similar group to his or her own and provides some indication as to whether or not the results can be generalized.

Next there should be some indication of the method/model of selection clearly stating any inclusion/exclusion criteria. If there is insufficient evidence that this has been carried out satisfactorily, then sample bias may affect the external validity (generalizability) of the study.

The report should also state whether randomization took place. In theory, all people should have an equal opportunity of being selected for the study. If the sample of the population is selected in a non-random manner, or is a convenience sample, then this too can lead to sample bias with the potential for incorrect inferences/conclusions to be made.

Any attrition or non-participation should have been documented, with reasons, as this may affect the credibility of the study, for example if people were dropping out because there had been breaches of confidentiality.

The above should enable the reader to determine the representativeness of the sample in relation to the target population and help determine its generalizability.

Additionally, when reading quantitative research reports the sample size should be considered. In general, large sample sizes are viewed as essential. However, a small sample size should not necessarily be viewed as bad, but it is important to be aware that it may affect the powers of statistical analysis.

The reader should also consider the setting in which the research was undertaken, as this has implications for external validity.

Data collection

The author should have fully described the instruments used to collect data, as this enables readers to replicate the study. In particular, the instruments utilized should relate to the operationalization of the concepts/variables. This enables the reader to determine whether they actually measure what the researcher intended them to measure and gives an indication of the internal validity of the study (the extent to which a test variable truthfully reflects the effects of a test variable).

Reliability and validity of the instruments are essential elements of the research process and if the instrument does not have face validity (is not accepted as a 'gold' standard) or has not been standardized, then the researcher should have taken steps to standardize it, otherwise questions will be asked. To do this, a pilot study should have been undertaken and any problems experienced reported along with any remedial action taken.

The design

The study design should facilitate the generation of unambiguous and meaningful results, and the following questions should be asked:

1 Is the researcher looking for causal effects of one variable (the independent variable) upon another (the dependent variable), in which case the study should be experimental in design?
2 Is the researcher looking for relationships between variables, in which case the design should be correlational?
3 Is the researcher trying to get an overview of current practice, attitudes, etc., in which case a survey has actually been undertaken?
4 Is the researcher looking at experience? If this is the case, it is probably qualitative research and different criteria should be used to critique the published paper.

In the first two cases, poor design can result in uncontrolled influences by extraneous variables (something outside the study that is not considered but may have affected the results) and in case 1, one could question if cause and effect can be proven with any degree of probability. In this case, a control group should have been used – without one it is difficult to estimate the extent of any effect, and they are particularly useful for controlling for any extraneous effects. However, at the same time the equivalence of the control and experimental groups is important. If they consist of markedly different individuals then this may introduce bias to the study and influence its internal validity (the extent to which measurement truthfully reflects the effects of a test variable) as much as if there was no control group.

Statistics

Tables and graphs should have been correctly tabulated and drawn, and should have adequate labelling to enable the reader to understand them. Complete summaries of all relevant findings should have been included.

Any statistical tests undertaken should have been done, bearing in mind that:

- they are appropriate for the level of data
- they are congruent with the research questions or hypotheses
- descriptive or inferential statistics are performed according to the rules.

Failure to follow the above may result in distortion of the findings, leading to inappropriate inferences. Never assume that calculations are correct. It is useful in the first instance to check for obvious errors and then, if sufficient information is available, recheck the results to ensure their accuracy.

It is also important to note whether or not the significance is reported and if so at what level. This will enable the reader to determine the probability that the results may, or may not, have occurred by chance.

Discussion

In this section, the researcher should be drawing inferences and interpreting the findings of the study. In essence, the author should be making sense of the analysis, bearing in mind the sampling procedures, practical constraints and data quality. Therefore the author should also be considering the strengths and limitations of the study and making recommendations as to how the research could be undertaken more rigorously if it were to be repeated.

Bearing in mind that the research began with a literature review and the development of a theoretical framework, this section should also consider the relationship of the knowledge developed during the research process to that which was already known.

Any deviations from the original intentions should be clearly outlined with reasons and justification given for any post-hoc analysis unrelated to the original research questions or hypotheses. Some papers may move focus without making it clear why. Therefore the reader may find that the findings and discussion do not relate to the original title/question and the study validity (does the study measure what it sets out to measure?) may be brought into question.

It is not just the statistical significance of the findings that is important, nurses also have to bear in mind the practical or clinical significance when deciding whether or not to use the results in practice. Also, the researcher should have added a note of caution about implementing the research in practice if there is no evidence that it can be repeated.

Presentation

Having critiqued the research report it may be useful to consider the presentation and style of its author(s). While it is important to undertake research in practice, it is equally important that the researcher has communicated the findings in such a way that a wide range of individuals can understand them. It follows then that the author(s) should avoid jargon wherever possible.

The report should demonstrate logical consistency and flow in such a way that the process undertaken is easily identifiable and replicable. Therefore the report should be structured and systematic, with headings and subheadings as appropriate.

Each section of the report should provide sufficient information for the reader to assess its credibility. If information is lacking, it follows that judgements cannot be made and the research cannot be used. However, one has to remember that for the sake of publication, strict word limits are often applied and this means that some information will be lost. Often the literature review is condensed and ethics only mentioned at the expense of analysis and discussion.

Qualitative research

Qualitative research is derived from different theoretical orientations to quantitative research but many people try to critique it using models usually applied to quantitative research. As a result, the research is often said to lack credibility. The following aims to highlight where differences in approach may be required.

An important point to make here is that because of the subjective and interpretative nature of qualitative research, the paper should be presented in such a way that the reader can see a rigorous process of data collection and analysis taking place. And, where necessary, it should demonstrate how the problems of researcher bias were overcome.

The literature review

There is some argument that a literature review should not be undertaken prior to a qualitative study as it may serve to bias the investigator during data collection and analysis. However, there is also an argument that it would be impossible to undertake a literature review and not have it in mind while the research is in progress. It may be that the author chooses to include a literature review to show how the work may have been influenced. In addition, a literature review may have been necessary to determine that there was a need for the research and in particular that a qualitative approach may cast a new light on the matter in hand.

The literature is often referred to after the presentation of findings with the purpose of justifying and explaining the concepts developed during the data analysis procedures.

The theoretical framework

Many authors argue that there should be no theoretical framework to guide qualitative studies because the framework should be developed from the results of data analysis. One view is that the framework would inhibit or limit the researcher's development of ideas and expression of issues that may need exploring. The advice therefore is that the researcher should put his or her knowledge of these issues to one side. However, another view is that it would be naive to claim that the researcher had no preconceptions about what the study would be about, because prior reading and experience cannot be put out of mind. In this case, the researcher should have made any influencing factors known to the reader, who can then assess whether or not the findings have been significantly biased. One way of doing this is for the researcher to present a conceptual framework.

The sample

Qualitative research does not require large numbers selected in a random manner. Such studies aim to describe experience and not collect numbers for statistical analysis. What is more important is that the sample has been drawn from a population in which there is some similarity of experience on which the researcher may draw in order to develop the study. So if the study was to examine the postoperative experience of women post-mastectomy, it follows that the sample should be made up of women who have undergone such surgery. However, there can still be inclusion and exclusion criteria, such as age, length of time postoperative, etc., so that the study becomes more focused. There is some debate about numbers within the literature, but a general view is that if the sample is homogenous then small numbers (8-10) are acceptable. However, the more heterogeneous a sample becomes, the wiser it is to choose larger numbers (up to 20). It is important that the researcher has justified the sample size, but bear in mind that in qualitative research the phenomenon of interest is more important than the sample size.

Data collection

Invariably the most frequently used form of data collection in qualitative research is the interview.

Structured interviews

Generally, these should not be used in qualitative research. They are similar in content to the questionnaires used in quantitative research and often result in the need for the researcher to classify and count numbers of responses to each question. This conflicts with qualitative philosophy.

Semi-structured interviews

These allow more freedom of response by the participants, but there can be a tendency for the researcher to undertake a counting exercise if he or she is not careful.

Unstructured interviews

These allow a much wider response from the participant and often result in a rich source of data necessary for qualitative analysis. However, it may be difficult to get a clear focus on the phenomenon being studied. In light of this, the researcher may have steered more towards semi-structured interviews, initially or after a couple of unstructured interviews when some light has been cast on the matter in question. The researcher should continue the interviews until no new data is found or the categories have become saturated. Failure to do so will result in a weak theory or descriptive accounts of experience with little substance.

Observation

Often the qualitative interviewer chooses to enter the setting under study and observe actions/interactions as a form of data collection. If this form of data collection has taken place, the researcher should have made explicit how he or she overcame the potential problem that their presence may have influenced the actions of those being observed.

Bias

Because of the subjective nature of data collection in qualitative research, the paper should contain some information about how the problem of bias in interpreting dialogue from interviews and observations of the subject in the setting was overcome.

Data analysis

It is important that the reader is able to judge the credibility of the findings by the rigour of the data analysis. The paper should include an explanation of the coding, categorization and development of concepts. This should obviously be reflective of the approach, i.e. grounded theory, phenomenology or ethnography. Data collection and analysis should occur concurrently to develop the emerging themes/ideas (as in grounded theory).

A more in-depth discussion of these issues can be found in texts specific to each methodology. The reader should be able to follow the process of analysis through rigorous description provided by the researcher; otherwise it would be difficult to judge the credibility of the findings.

Presentation of findings

While qualitative research does not result in statistical tables, it does present large numbers of data that need to be expressed in a succinct manner. This is usually done in two ways:

*   First, a diagram or model is developed. This should be clear and understandable, identifying the concepts and their inter-relationships where appropriate.
*   The model should be accompanied by an interesting and stimulating story that should also be credible. This is often done

through discussion of the concepts and categories and their inter-relationships, which should have been supported in two ways.

Quotes from participants

Quotes from participants are frequently used to show data that supports the emergent concepts. They should relate to the concept and demonstrate that what is being said has been interpreted appropriately by the researcher and accurately conveys the meaning of what has been said. It is important that the researcher has maintained the client's anonymity, and not used quotes from which others could potentially identify the individual being quoted.

The literature

After presentung the findings, the interpretations of interview data can be given further substance by examining them in relation to the published literature. If this is carried out before the start of the study it can bias the results, but done afterwards it gives the researcher a chance to demonstrate where the differences and similarities lie and perhaps consider further why this may be so. Some researchers may have accessed the literature during data collection; this is called theoretical sampling and is used to further develop emergent concepts.

It is important that this part of the research paper is not a simple description containing endless lists of quotes from interview transcripts and/or the literature. It should be analytical and demonstrate abstracting of the identified concepts through interpretation of data.

Action point
- Go back to your research papers and see if they missed anything out.
- Was it clear and jargon-free?
- And most importantly, will it make you reconsider your practice?

Summary

This chapter should enable you to examine critically the process by which research has been undertaken, and help you judge whether or not it can be used in clinical practice. However, the information provided is in no way exhaustive and should be read in conjunction with the other chapters of this book and the texts listed below.

References

Davies S (1998) Reviewing and interpreting research: identifying implications for practice. In Crookes PA, Davies S (eds) Research into Practice. London: Ballière Tindall/RCN.

Hibbert C, Crookes P (1998) Accessing sources of knowledge. In Crookes PA, Davies S (eds) Research into Practice. London: Ballière Tindall/RCN.

Kneale J, Knight C (1997) Do orthopaedic nurses have an effect on the quality of patient care? Journal of Orthopaedic Nursing 1(1): 115-17.

Lewis DM, Barnes C (1997) Critiquing the research literature. In Smith PM (ed) Research Mindedness for Practice: an interactive approach for healthcare. London: Churchill Livingstone.

Polgar S, Thomas SA (1995) Introduction to Research in the Health Sciences. London: Churchill Livingstone.

Polit DF, Hungler DP (1997) Critiquing research reports. In The Essentials of Nursing Research: methods, appraisal and utilisation, 4th edn. London: Lipincott.

Santy J, Kneale J (1998) Critiquing quantitative research. Journal of Orthopaedic Nursing 2(2): 77-83.

Further reading

DePoy E, Gitlin LN (1993) Introduction to Research: multiple strategies for health and human sciences. St Louis, MO: Mosby.

Hicks CM (1990) Research and Statistics: a practical introduction for nurses. London: Prentice Hall.

Holloway I, Wheeler S (1996) Qualitative Research for Nurses. London: Blackwell.

Marshall C, Rossman GB (1995) Designing Qualitative Research, 2nd edn. London: Sage.

Morse J (1994) Qualitative Health Research. London: Sage.

CHAPTER FIVE

Exploring and overcoming the barriers to research utilization: strengthening evidence-based care

GENE W MARSH

Introduction

There are many different ways of implementing research findings in the clinical setting. However, for nurses, the emphasis is on basing the decisions about the care they provide to patients on current research findings. The process of using research findings to guide clinical decision making is a major factor in providing evidence-based care. Evidence-based practice, or the process of providing evidence-based care, is defined as follows:

> The conscientious, explicit, and judicious use of current best evidence, based on systematic review of all available evidence – including patient-reported, clinician-observed and research derived evidence – in making and carrying out decisions about the care of individual patients. The best available evidence, moderated by patient circumstances and preferences is applied to improve the quality of clinical judgements (McKibbon et al. 1995; National Centre for Clinical Audit 1997).

One can deduce from this definition that an evidence-based nursing care decision may be derived from several sources of information, including current accepted practice, patient preferences, specific patient circumstances, information reported by colleagues, practice guidelines and organizational policy. When there are no research findings it is necessary to draw on these other sources of information to reach the best nursing care decision. For example, how would you decide what to do for a postoperative patient who has been sleep-deprived due to pain and is finally sleeping soundly but is scheduled to be turned? Which nursing action would take priority, promoting sleep and pain relief, or promoting oxygen diffusion in the lungs? How would you make this decision? Would you simply follow the doctor's orders? Would you need other information such as the patient's age, respiratory status, vital signs, history of pulmonary conditions, knowledge of whether or not the patient is a smoker, degree of pain when awake, duration and type of surgical procedure? Or in the case of a primary care patient who has chronic arthritis in both knees, would you get the GP to prescribe something stronger for pain relief, explore the patient's home circumstances, finding out if there are any circumstances that might be causing extra pain, or consider acupuncture or complementary therapies? Nurses who provide evidence-based care must critically appraise the available evidence that will promote positive health outcomes for patients.

Action point

- Think what steps you might take with a patient of yours.
- What data do you build up to enhance the nursing skills you can provide?

Although nurse researchers are continuing to generate scientific evidence on which to base care decisions, the diffusion of research findings into clinical practice is still lagging far behind their generation. Hunt (1981) described five reasons why nurses do not use research findings:

- Nurses are unaware of the research findings.
- They do not understand them.
- They do not believe what the findings indicate.
- They do not know how to apply them.
- They are not allowed to use them.

Hunt herself questions the progress we have made in 15 years of attempting to conquer these barriers to research utilization (Hunt

1996). She also attributed the failure of nurses to utilize research findings to factors other than individual nurse characteristics, such as structures and processes of healthcare organizations, and characteristics of the nursing research itself (Hunt 1981).

Implementing research in clinical settings is a complex process and necessitates understanding:

- the relationship between the healthcare system and the generation of nursing knowledge for practice, or the structure and process that underlies the research culture
- the process of planning and implementing change by utilizing an established change framework
- the identification of barriers that prevent nurses from utilizing research findings in practice
- the structures and processes that can potentially enable, influence and stimulate an evidence-based work culture. These four areas comprise the focus of this chapter.

The relationship between healthcare systems and the generation of nursing knowledge

Although research utilization and evidence-based care are receiving increasing global attention, much of the background information on research utilization originates from the US. It is worth examining how US nursing has strengthened its national infrastructure in carefully executed stages, often through the combined efforts of nurse leaders in research, education and practice working together to influence policy development which is supportive to knowledge development and practice implementation.

Research utilization in the US

It is recognized in the US that there must be a national infrastructure along with resources that support expansion of nursing knowledge (Hinshaw 1999). Federal involvement in nursing research began in 1946, with the establishment of the Division of Nursing, and the funding of nursing research in 1955. In 1960, a restructured Division of Nursing was created within the Health Resources and Services

Administration (HRSA). Clinical training was strengthened through educational grants, and there was continud funding for research. In the 1970s, two Division of Nursing-funded projects focused on the process of transferring research findings into clinical practice settings. They are frequently cited in the British literature (Closs & Cheater 1994; Lacy 1994; McDonnell 1998).

Research utilization projects in the US

The US Division of Nursing under the federal government funded the Western Institute for Communication in Higher Education (WICHE) project directed by Krueger (Krueger et al. 1978). The purpose of the project was to increase research activities in nursing in western US. The WICHE project involved developing a model of research utilization based on Havelock's linker system theory (Havelock and Havelock 1973), and linked nursing resources with users of nursing research in clinical settings.

From 1975 to 1980, the Division of Nursing funded the Conduct and Utilization of Research in Nursing (CURN) project (Horsley et al. 1978). This project envisioned research utilization as an organizational process rather than an individual professional responsibility and it was also evaluated at the organizational level. The project utilized Rogers's innovation diffusion theory (Rogers 1962) and resulted in the development of research-based clinical protocols that were tested in clinical trials and evaluated for effectiveness. Ten areas were considered to have sufficient quality research to warrant implementation (CURN Project 1981-82). The process utilizes a clinical effectiveness framework and resulted in increased research-based practice at the organizational level. Both the WICHE and the CURN projects demonstrate commitment from the federal level to foster the necessary communication and transfer of knowledge between researchers and practicing nurses.

National Institute for Nursing Research (NINR)

The establishment of the National Centre for Nursing Research (NCNR) at the National Institutes of Health (NIH) in 1986 (Hinshaw 1999) stimulated rapid growth in nursing research and research traditions within the US. The NCNR was redesignated as the National Institute of Nursing Research (NINR) in 1993. Many national nursing organizations, the nation's community of nurse scholars and the Division of Nursing are credited with providing the direction and support necessary for this significant landmark in nursing's history. The mission of the NINR is to 'facilitate national programs of nursing research and promote excellence in knowledge base developed for the profession' (US Department of Health and Human Services 2000).

The NCNR/NINR was responsible for developing the National Nursing Research Agenda. Two phases of the National Nursing Research Agenda identified the major health issues that nursing could influence given a solid base of research (Bloch 1990; Hinshaw 1999). The first phase focused on selected research priorities that would yield in-depth research in specific clinical areas of study, such as long-term care of older persons and prevention and care of individuals with HIV infection. The findings were instrumental in building nursing science and enriching clinical practice (Hinshaw et al. 1988). The second priority area focused on research training and career development. Funding awards were established to support study and career development of researchers (Hinshaw et al. 1988).

Agency for Health Care Policy Research (AHCPR)

In 1989, another US government agency, the Agency for Health Care Policy Research (AHCPR), convened panels of expert healthcare providers and researchers to review and summarize research, and develop clinical practice guidelines. Initially guidelines were developed in 18 areas, such as acute pain management and urinary incontinence. The purpose of the guidelines is to promote quality healthcare that is based on best evidence and will improve patient outcomes.

The Division of Nursing, NINR and AHCPR have all been instrumental in providing an infrastructure as well as necessary resources for enriching the development of nursing science, which will inform practice in priority areas. Information about the NINR and the AHCPR guidelines may be found on the NIH website (http://www.nih.gov).

Research utilization in the UK

> **Action point**
>
> - Where do you think we are in research utilization in the UK?
> - What assistance is there that you know of that can help you implement research in your workplace, hospital trust or PCG?

As recently as 1994, Closs and Cheater stated that the NHS appears to undervalue research and as a result it is not surprising that the appropriate and successful utilization of nursing research poses considerable problems. While this statement may capture the feelings of some, others would argue that the NHS has been promoting an evidence-based culture for many years.

NHS research and development strategy

The NHS research and development strategy was published in 1991 (DoH 1991) and stressed the objective that care in the NHS should be based on research relevant to improving the health of the nation. Subsequent publications of government policy expressed the expectation that patient care should be evidence-based.

In 1993, the more in-depth strategy *Research for Health* was published. This emphasized the need to ensure that beneficial findings from research are translated into practice (DoH 1993; Read 1998). *The Culyer Report* (Culyer 1994) and implementation plans have resulted in research activity at the trust and regional level. Changes in funding mechanisms should result in better support for non-medical health research and research resources (Read 1998), such as educational development of nurses preparing to use research findings in practice.

The expectation that nursing care should be evidence-based is emphasized within three additional publications of government policy: *The New NHS: modern, dependable* (DoH 1997), *A First Class*

Service: quality in the new NHS (DoH, 1998) and *Making a Difference* (DoH 1999). Together these policy papers set the course for 'services and treatment across the NHS that are based on the best evidence of what does and does not work and what provides the best value for money' (DoH 1997). The most recent of the policy papers, *Making a Difference* (DoH 1999), is directed towards nurses', midwives' and health visitors' contributions to healthcare. Two points of reference about research emphasize the need to provide care that is guided by best evidence. The first focuses on the need to strengthen nurses' skill for interpreting and appraising research findings. The second high-lights forthcoming strategies.

- Practice needs to be evidence-based. Research evidence will be rigorously assessed and made accessible. Nurses, midwives and health visitors need better research appraisal skills to translate research findings into practice.
- A strategy to influence the research and development agenda, to strengthen the capacity to undertake nursing, midwifery and health visiting research, and to use research to support a nursing midwifery and health visiting practice will be developed (DoH 1999).

Nurses in clinical practice, research, administrative and educational positions commonly agree that patient care must be evidence-based. Providing care that is evidence-based is one way that we implement research findings in clinical settings. An underlying assumption of evidence-based care is that it will stimulate more positive patient and system outcomes. This also translates into the provision of clinically effective care, or care that is high in quality and cost-effective in relation to the use of human and material resources. For example, care that is high in quality should not be delivered at the expense of extending the length of stay in acute facilities, as this prevents or delays others from receiving timely, quality care.

Both the US and the UK have acknowledged the importance of creating a culture that delivers evidence-based care. Both have developed strategies and plans for changing their research and practice cultures. Working through the NINR, the US has funded researchers, systematically identified the priority problems of relevance and directed research efforts towards building science to address these problems. Results have been published and disseminated. Partnerships have been formed with clinicians, educators and nurse executives to stimulate the uptake of research findings in the practice arena. Within the UK, NHS policy papers have presented strategies articulating the importance of evidence-based care and the critical need for practitioners who have sufficient knowledge and skill to implement research findings. Unfortunately, the funding resources for implementing these strategies in the UK lag far behind those of the US. In addition, the number of nurses who have been educated to conduct research is limited (Hicks 1995). Yet, without the support of the NHS infrastructure, progress in research utilization would be far more problematic.

Planning and implementing change

Before change can take place, a well-developed plan must be created. There are many theories, frameworks and models available for planning change. Examples of change theories and frameworks that have guided implementing changes in nurses' utilization of research findings include:

Havelock's linker system theory (Havelock and Havelock 1973)

- Lewin's (1951) Force Field Analysis
- Rogers's (1995) Innovation Diffusion Theory.

Full references to these theories, frameworks and models are given at the end of the chapter. However, Rogers's (1995) Innovation Diffusion Theory is given greater attention here.

Everett M Rogers is a professor and chair of the Department of Communication and Journalism at the University of New Mexico. His Innovation Diffusion Theory first appeared in 1962 and has undergone three revisions (Rogers and Shoemaker 1971; Rogers 1983, 1995). Rogers (1995, p 10) defines diffusion as the process by which an innovation is communicated through certain channels over time among the members of a social system. 'Innovation', 'communication channels', 'time' and 'social system' comprise the elements or building blocks of the theory. Rogers describes the 'innovation' as a new idea, practice or object. In the change discussed in this chapter, evidence-based nursing practice is the innovation.

'Communication channels' are the means by which a message is transmitted from one individual to another (Rogers 1995). The third element is 'time' and it characterizes how long it may take individuals, or other decision-making units such as organizations, to go through the steps of the innovative-decision process (Rogers 1995). 'Social system', the fourth element, is defined as a set of interrelated units that are engaged in joint problem solving to accomplish a common goal (Rogers 1995). An NHS trust with the goal of providing quality healthcare exemplifies a social system. But, individuals, informal groups and organizational subsystems may also comprise social systems.

According to Rogers (1995, p 20) the innovation-decision process consists of five steps:

- knowledge
- persuasion
- decision
- implementation
- confirmation.

Knowledge occurs when an individual gains an understanding about the innovation. Persuasion refers to the individual or organization forming a positive attitude toward the innovation. Decision is the result of an individual or organization taking action and making a choice to accept or reject the innovation. Implementation occurs when the individual or organization puts the innovation to use. Confirmation occurs when an individual seeks reinforcement about an innovation-decision that has been made.

Applied to an individual staff nurse named Jane, the innovation-decision process might occur in the following manner. First, Jane, out of her own curiosity or at the suggestion of her manager, may attend a class or workshop about evidence-based practice. She may come away from the workshop having enjoyed the study leave and having time to reflect on her practice. Jane's thoughts are positive, and she considers that evidence-based practice would be a good thing for patients, even though it will require more work and more of her time. She considers that the extra time may result in valuable improvements in patient care and decides that the next time she has a question about her own practice she will attempt to find a research article suggesting the method for administering patient care. When a question arises about the best way to position a confused elderly patient, Jane finds a research article that discusses levels of environmental stimulation that may improve orientation in the elderly patient, such as positioning him facing towards the centre of the room rather than towards the wall. She shows the article to her nurse manager and together they convene a short staff meeting to communicate the findings to the other nurses. The nurses discuss the benefits of the nursing care intervention, and several indicate they are going to try it and will report back to the group. Jane is convinced that providing evidence-based practice has positive results and she continues to investigate her questions. Not only has she begun to modify her own behaviour, but she has also positively influenced her colleagues. She has become an opinion leader. Opinion leaders are those individuals who are able to influence other individuals' attitudes or behaviour informally in a desired way with relative frequency (Rogers 1995).

Rogers categorizes adopters of an innovation into five groups characterized by the rate of time it takes the group to accomplish the steps of the innovation-decision process. The categories are defined as:

- *innovators*, the most venturesome members of the social system
- *early adopters*, well-integrated members of the social system who may also function as opinion leaders
- *early majority*, the largest and most deliberate group of members in the social system, likely to change but not to lead
- *late majority*, individuals who are more sceptical and adopt new ideas after the average member of the system
- *laggards*, the most traditional, resistant and last members to adopt a new idea (Rogers 1995).

Rogers utilizes a normal distribution to depict the continuous diffusion process across all member categories of a social system or organization. The rate of adoption of an innovation is the relative speed with which an innovation, such as evidence-based practice, is adopted by members of the social system (Rogers 1995).

Action point

- Think about the people you work with in the surgery or ward. Can you begin to identify any of the types that Rogers identified?
- Can you think of any ways you might help win them over to aid you in implementing change?

Understanding the innovation-diffusion process and the categories of members that comprise an organization or social system can be critical in planning change. A grasp of this important information will enable a change agent to know when and to whom successful change strategies should be targeted.

Identifying barriers to research utilization

Just as the NHS has identified the necessity of ensuring that patient care is evidence-based, local trusts and PCGs are exploring, identifying and developing strategies to address barriers to research utilization at the local area. Such studies are useful in forming the foundation for subsequent changes that may influence the local research culture (Dunn et al. 1998; Nolan et al. 1998; Marsh et al. 1999). Several studies have utilized the Barriers to Research Utilisation Scale (Funk et al. 1991a,b) to carry out an initial assessment of their organizational settings.

The Barriers to Research Utilization Scale (Barriers Scale) has been used in the US and the UK for the past several years to measure the magnitude and scope of perceived barriers that prevent nurses from using research findings to guide clinical decision making and practice. The rationale exists that if barriers can be adequately identified and measured, strategies to overcome identified barriers can then be implemented in practice settings, thus improving patient care by ensuring that it is guided by current research findings.

The 29-item Barriers Scale was developed in the US by Funk, Champagne, Wiese and Tournquist (1991a,b). Its content was identified and developed from the literature, from the CURN project and from informal data collected from nurses (Crane et al. 1977; Funk et al. 1991b).

Funk et al.'s (1991a) scale consists of four subscales that are consistent with Rogers's (1995) theory. Funk et al. (1991a) represent Rogers's communication channels as the presentation of the research, including its accessibility. Rogers's innovation is characterized by Funk et al. (1991a) as the characteristics of the research itself. They represent Rogers's time dimension, or characteristics of the adopter of the research, with the nurse. Characteristics such as the nurse's research values, skills, awareness and the time involved to move through the process of adopting the research innovation are included. The final Barrier's subscale, organisational setting, corresponds to Rogers's (1995) social system.

Nolan et al. (1998) revised the language of the Barriers Scale to yield a scale that would contain language that was more easily recognized by UK nurses, or a scale that was more UK-friendly. In a subsequent study, Marsh et al. (1999) found that the subscales identified by Funk et al. (1991a,b) were not upheld when the scale was used with samples of UK nurses. They advocate using the revised scale for identifying and ranking individual barriers within an organizational or clinical setting, but not for making interpretations from the broader subscales (Marsh et al. 1999).

Examining structures and processes that may stimulate an evidence-based work culture

But what is the next step? What happens once national policy dictates that research findings should be the basis for providing evidence-based care? We know that merging the agendas of nursing research and nursing practice means building the bridge that spans the research practice gap, unites the two and creates a culture of practice that allows best evidence to be communicated in understandable ways. We know that it will take the support of administrators, researchers, educators and practitioners working together to identify the barriers to research utilization and to influence the uptake of research findings into professional practice by individual nurses. Even if one understands the change process and the necessary steps for an innovation to be accepted and implemented, how can a culture actually be changed?

Closs and Cheater (1994) suggest that there are three prerequisites for successful research utilization:

- wide-ranging support from governmental bodies, managers and peers
- a positive research culture
- interest from those who have the potential to utilize findings in practice.

This is another way of saying that support must exist at the government and policy level, the organizational or trust level, and the individual or practitioner level. In addition, each existing culture may have different characteristics and different barriers to research utilization. To illustrate how complex cultural change can be systematically implemented, the experience of one large NHS trust will be the focus of the remainder of this chapter.

Changing the research utilization culture: a case study

The NHS document *A First Class Service* (DoH 1998) and preceding papers foretold the coming of clinical governance:

> Clinical governance is a framework through which NHS organisations are accountable for continuously improving the quality of their services and safeguarding high standards of care by creating an environment in which excellence in clinical care will flourish.

Quality improvement activities that are outlined in the document state that evidence-based practice must be supported and applied routinely in everyday practice. The implications are not just for medicine, but for all care providers within the NHS.

Strengthening organizational support

The director of nursing for the Central Sheffield University Hospitals Trust (CSUH) envisioned that the structure of nursing and midwifery care delivery would need to change. Evidence-based practice needed to be assured, but other changes would be necessary to promote continuing professional development and lifelong learning as investments in the quality of patient care and health outcomes. She envisioned that nurses would need to value their organization and become empowered in shaping their own futures and ability to influence the continuous provision of quality care. Not all trusts are fortunate in having such a forward-looking director of nursing who believes in revitalizing the nursing and midwifery organizational structure to create the support necessary for cultural change.

Achieving shared governance would require the creation of many new partnerships. First, the director of nursing began introducing the idea of a shared governance nursing structure within the trust. Shared governance is an innovative approach for building a professional and empowered nursing organization within a healthcare system. Shared governance relies on the principles of partnership, equity, accountability and ownership (Porter-O'Grady 1996). A full discussion of shared governance is not within the scope of this chapter. However, there are many publications, especially those authored by Timothy Porter-O'Grady, which present a detailed explanation of shared governance as well as methods of implementation and evaluation.

Creating the research-practice partnership

Although the envisioned changes were far-reaching, only the changes related to promoting evidence-based practice will be discussed in this chapter. The director of nursing recognized the need to create a research-practice partnership to help in bridging the research-practice gap. The University of Sheffield and the CSUH jointly funded a professor of acute and critical care nursing to serve as the trust's nursing research lead and oversee the diffusion of evidence-based practice among the many directorates of the trust.

Identifying the barriers to research utilization

The professor of acute and critical care nursing designed and conducted an initial descriptive study to identify and describe the perceived barriers to research utilization perceived by nurses and midwives within the CSUH. The data-collection instrument used for the study was the revised Barriers Scale (Nolan et al. 1998; Marsh et al. 1999). During one month in 1998, 1509 Barriers instruments were sent to all nurses and midwives within the trust. The response rate was modest, 37.3%, but was a true representation of the CSUH workforce.

Ranking the barriers

The ranking of barriers by percentage of respondents reporting them as 'a moderate or great barrier' is depicted in Table 5.1. Six of

Table 5.1 Ranked barriers by percentage of respondents reporting item as a moderate or great barrier to research utilization

Rank	Barrier	% reporting moderate or great barrier	Frequency/ number of valid responses
1	There is insufficient time at work to implement new ideas	82.0	446/544
2	Resources are inadequate for implementation	79.7	429/538
3	The statistics are difficult to understand	75.8	413/545
4	The nurse does not feel that she/he has enough authority to change patient care procedures	73.8	399/541
5	The relevant research literature is not available in one place	71.1	382/537
6	Doctors will not co-operate with implementation	71.0	373/525
7	The nurse does not have time to read research	70.8	385/544
8	The research is not easy to read and understand	65.8	356/541
9	Other staff are not supportive of implementation	62.6	336/537
10	The nurse does not know what research is available	62.5	340/544
11	Implications for changing practice are not made clear	59.6	322/540
12	The nurse does not feel able to read the research critically or evaluate it	58.1	313/539
13	The amount of research information available is overwhelming	57.9	308/532
14	The research findings are only based on a one-off study	51.8	261/503
15	It is difficult to find knowledgeable colleagues with whom to discuss the research	50.0	268/536
16	The literature reports conflicting results	48.7	246/505
17	The nurse is uncertain whether to believe the results of the research	48.7	260/534
18	Research reports/articles are not readily available	48.0	262/546
19	Managers will not allow implementation	46.2	240/520
20	Nurses do not feel results apply to their own settings	45.7	243/532
21	Research reports/articles are not published fast enough	44.7	211/472
22	The research methods used are inadequate	42.8	198/463
23	The nurse is unwilling to change/try new ideas	41.0	223/544
24	Nurses see little benefit to themselves in implementing research results	37.8	202/535
25	The nurse feels the benefits of changing practice will be minimal	37.1	195/525
26	The research is not relevant to the nurse's practice	34.0	180/530
27	The conclusions drawn from the research are not supported by the findings	28.1	135/481
28	There is no written evidence of the need to change practice	25.6	134/523
29	The nurse does not see the value of research for practice	19.6	106/541

the top ten barriers were related to the perceptions about the organizational setting, three of the top ten barriers revealed perceptions that research findings either lacked clarity for future implementation or were unavailable or difficult to access. One of the top ten barriers was related to perceptions that users of the research were not confident or were unknowing about the utilization of research findings.

Extending organizational support

While the barriers study was being conducted, the director of nursing was extending the development of organizational support to include nurse managers. Time-outs were held and creative group sessions ensued. Managers worked through issues and concerns about the new shared governance structure. They also began owning and shaping the dynamic structure that would eventually evolve. Working collaboratively as what Rogers refers to as 'innovators', the nurse managers, director of nursing and professor of acute and critical care nursing began shaping plans for an Evidence-based Council that would represent each directorate and would accept the challenge to create an evidence-based nursing practice culture.

Launching the Evidence-based Council

The Evidence-based Council was developed to address the identified barriers to research utilization within the trust and to promote the necessary positive cultural changes that would support evidence-based nursing practice. Council membership was comprised of a director, deputy director and members representing the nursing or midwifery research lead for each directorate. Large directorates were designated two members. Members will eventually be elected to the council by their nurse colleagues within each directorate. Initially, however, they were selected because of their commitment to the principles of evidence-based practice and to the organization. In other words, they fulfilled Rogers's (1995) definition of 'opinion leaders' and would be key to the diffusion of new ideas within their directorates. The purposes of the Evidence-based Council are presented in Table 5.2.

Table 5.2 Purposes of the Evidence-based Council

- To develop, implement, support and evaluate processes within and between directorates that will stimulate nursing practice based on best available evidence
- To educate nurses, midwives and their colleagues in the process of gathering, systematically reviewing and judging the clinical adequacy of available evidence for guiding nursing practice
- To participate in changing, documenting and evaluating practice protocols, and monitor practice changes intended to improve patient outcomes of nursing care
- To influence nursing clinical governance at the directorate level by initiating, supporting and sustaining evidence-based nursing practice

---

Initially, the council established four goals and strategies for achieving each goal. The goals were:

- To formalize the mission of the Evidence-based Council and establish the operational structure and guidelines.
- To create an environment conducive to the practice of evidence-based nursing and midwifery and the conduct of nursing research.
- To conduct the process of systematic review of evidence within each directorate.
- To develop a database and tracking system of the products of scholarly achievement among nurses and midwives across all directorates.

The purposes of the council were consistent with the need to create cultural change within the organization while the goals and accompanying strategies reflected its intent to address barriers to research utilization.

Strengthening opinion leader skills

The strength of the opinion leaders in influencing change at the directorate level was critical to creating an evidence-based nursing practice culture. To assure that opinion leaders (council members) would feel knowledgeable and confident in their new roles, the professor of nursing designed, developed and facilitated a research awareness course that addressed specific nurse-related barriers to research utilization as well as individual needs of council members. The course was offered over four full days, and the director of nursing funded replacement personnel for each directorate so that council members could be freed of daily responsibilities and focus on the course. Course content included sessions on development of research questions for systematic review, research design and methodology, searching for evidence in electronic databases, developing critical appraisal skills, starting a journal club and becoming a change agent.

The council's effectiveness in changing the nursing and midwifery research culture has only been evaluated in the formative stages. However, all of the first-year goals have been achieved and strategies have been enacted to systematically manage identified barriers. For example, the research awareness course strengthened opinion leaders' confidence and skill in accessing and appraising evidence for practice. Opinion leaders plan to mentor colleagues within their directorates in skills such as gathering, reviewing and critically evaluating and determining what constitutes best evidence. Some directorates have successfully implemented directorate research councils and journal clubs. Each council member, working collaboratively with clinical colleagues, has identified a clinical question for which evidence will be gathered and reviewed to evaluate best practice. Recognizing that sources of evidence for nursing are much broader than evidence derived from RCTs alone, council members have also developed a trust-wide methodology for gathering and reviewing nursing evidence and are planning to publish their model.

Access to research findings was identified as a major barrier to creating an evidence-based culture. The council was tenacious and assertive in improving access for all nurses in the trust. As a result, the trust purchased computer hardware and software that will facilitate 24-hour nursing access to research databases and the Internet for each council member. Access for other directorate nursing staff will be progressively expanded. Library access and holdings are currently being evaluated for adequacy in meeting the growing needs of nurses and midwives. There is increasing acceptance of nurses being able to access research and patient care information during scheduled work hours.

Although the organization has become more supportive of an evidence-based culture for nursing practice, diffusing change into the organization requires more than the support of the director of nursing, nurse managers and Evidence-based Council members.

Therefore, nursing is also represented on the multidisciplinary committees of the trust including the Research Management Committee, the Research Education Forum and multidisciplinary directorate research committees. Presentations about the council's mission have been made to all nurses in the trust as well as the trust executives.

With each success, council member confidence and commitment is reinforced. Employing a framework to guide the change process has helped council members to realistically pace themselves and the rate of change within their directorates. Mutual support among council members has mediated the discouragement individuals can feel when plans fail to materialize as expected. However, it is clear that the trust's nursing and midwifery opinion leaders are involved and committed in the process of changing the culture in which patient care is delivered. Change is valued and the members have achieved a growing sense of self-efficacy in facilitating change. Quite possibly after an initial 18 months of effort, the 'early majority' is beginning to move in a positive direction.

Action point

- Can you think of ways that the above example could be adapted to your own work place?
- Can you see ways that you might influence colleagues, such as GPs, doctors, managers, etc., by using change management approaches?

Conclusion

This chapter has illustrated that creating change that will facilitate research utilization by nurses or stimulating an evidence-based nursing practice culture may be initiated by national public policy. However, creating change at the organizational or trust level, the directorate level and individual level requires careful identification of the barriers that impede the uptake of research findings in practice. Strategies for overcoming barriers must then be planned and implemented. Organizational support is essential in fostering and facilitating the change process. In addition, nurses must value and own the plans for creating a new culture for evidence-based practice. One structure for creating cultural change is shared governance. However, transferring the change process from the organizational to the directorate level also requires the identification of knowledgeable and committed change agents or 'opinion leaders', who can painstakingly support one another, shape and strengthen their own professional development and leadership skills, and influence the infusion of change to a broader group of colleagues, the 'early majority'.

References

Bloch D (1990) Strategies for setting and implementing the National Center for Nursing Research priorities. Applied Nursing Research 3(1): 2-6.

Closs SJ and Cheater FM (1994) Utilization of nursing research: culture, interest and support. Journal of Advanced Nursing 19: 762-73.

Conduct and Utilization of Research in Nursing (CURN) Project (1981-82) Using Research to Improve Nursing Practice (series of clinical protocols). New York: Grune & Stratton.

Crane J, Pelz D, Horsley JA (1977) CURN Project Research Utilization Questionnaire. Ann Arbor, MI: Conduct and Utilization of Research in Nursing Project, School of Nursing, University of Michigan.

Culyer AJ (chair) (1994) Taskforce on Research and Development in the NHS. Supporting Research and Development in the NHS. London: HMSO.

Department of Health (1991) Research for Health: a research and development strategy for the NHS. London: HMSO.

Department of Health (1993) Research for Health. London: HMSO.

Department of Health (1997) The New NHS: modern, dependable. London: The Stationery Office.

Department of Health (1998) A First Class Service: quality in the new NHS. London: The Stationery Office.

Department of Health (1999) Making a Difference. London: The Stationery Office.

Dunn V, Crichton N, Roe B, Seers K, Williams K (1998) Using research for practice: a UK experience of the barriers scale. Journal of Advanced Nursing 26: 1203-10.

Funk SG, Champagne MT, Wiese RA, Tornquist EM (1991a) Barriers to using research findings in practice: the clinician's perspective. Applied Nursing Research 4(2): 90-5.

Funk SG, Champagne MT, Wiese RA, Tornquist EM (1991b) Barriers: the barriers to research utilization scale. Applied Nursing Research 4(1): 39-45.

Hicks C (1995) The shortfall in published research: a study of nurses' research and publication activities. Journal of Advanced Nursing 21: 594-604.

Havelock RG, Havelock MC (1973). Training for Change Agents: a guide to the design of training programs in education and other fields. Ann Arbor, MI: Center for Research on Utilization of Scientific Knowledge, Institute for Social Research, University of Michigan.

Hinshaw AS (1999) Evolving nursing research traditions. In Hinshaw AS et al. (eds) Handbook of Clinical Nursing Research. London: Sage, pp 19-30.

Hinshaw AS, Heinrich J, Bloch D (1988) Evolving clinical nursing research priorities: a national endeavor. Journal of Professional Nursing 4(6): 398, 458-9.

Horsley JA, Crane J, Bingle JD (1978) Research utilization as an organizational process. Journal of Nursing Administration 8(7): 4-6.

Hunt J (1981) Indications for nursing practice: the use of research findings. Journal of Advanced Nursing 6: 189-94.

Hunt J (1996) Barriers to research utilisation. Journal of Advanced Nursing 23(3): 423-5.

Krueger J, Nelson A, Wolanin MO (1978) Nursing Research Development Collaboration, and Utilization. Germantown, MD: Aspen Systems.

Lacy AE (1994) Research utilization in nursing practice – a pilot study. Journal of Advanced Nursing 19: 987-95.

Lewin K (1951) Cited in Lancaster J, Lancaster L (eds) Concepts for Advanced Nursing Practice: the nurse as change agent. St Louis, MO: Mosby.

Marsh GW, Nolan M, Hopkins S (1999) Testing the Revised Barriers to Research Utilisation Scale for use in the United Kingdom. Proceedings of the 1999 RCN Annual Nursing Research Conference held at Keele University. London: Royal College of Nursing.

McDonnell A (1998) Factors which may inhibit the utilization of research finidngs in practice – and some solutions In Crookes PC, Davies S (eds) Research into Practice, pp 259-80. Edinburgh: Baillière Tindall.

McKibbon KA, Wilcznski N, Hayward RS (1995) The medical literature as a resource for health care practice. Journal of American Society for Information Science 46: 737-42.

National Centre for Clinical Audit (1997) Glossary of Terms Used in NCCA Criteria for Clinical Audit. London: NCCA.

Nolan M, Morgan L, Curran M, Clayton J, Gerrish K, Parker K (1998) Evidence-based care: can we overcome the barriers? British Journal of Nursing 7(20): 1273-8.

Porter-O'Grady T (1996) Multidisciplinary shared governance: the next step. Seminars for Nurse Managers 4(1): 43-8.

Read S (1998) The context of nursing and health care research. In Crookes PC, Davies S (eds) Research into Practice, pp 23-54. Edinburgh, Baillière Tindall.

Rogers E (1962) Diffusion of Innovations. New York: The Free Press.

Rogers EM (1983) Diffusion of Innovations, 3rd edn. New York: The Free Press.

Rogers E (1995) Diffusion of Innovations, 4th edn. New York: The Free Press.

Rogers E, Shoemaker FF (1971) Communications of Innovations: a cross-cultural approach. New York: The Free Press.

Stetler C (1994) Refinement of the Stetler/Marram model for application of research findings to practice. Nursing Outlook 42(1): 15-25.

US Department of Health and Human Services (USDHHS), National Institutes of Health, National Institute of Nursing Research (2000) Website www.nih.gov/ninr/about.html

The local and national context of research: using research evidence to make quality improvements in healthcare

JANE HADDOCK

Introduction

The need to base healthcare on evidence that it has demonstrated both clinical and cost-effectiveness has never been greater. The impetus from practitioners has arisen from a growing realization, through questioning and reflection, that comparatively little is known about the effectiveness and efficiency of everyday practice. When evidence has been available it has been difficult to find, understand or use in terms of changing existing practice and persuading others to do so (Godlee 1998).

From the perspective of those who manage the NHS, evidence from epidemiological studies has highlighted wide variations in healthcare practice in both the process of service delivery and the outcomes of healthcare (DoH 1997). This also supports the notion that knowledge generated from healthcare research is not reaching practitioners or patients in a timely, systematic way.

As new technology, skills and knowledge are discovered, patients can more readily access information through the media and information technology such as the Internet, increasing their expectations of healthcare. This in turn raises the expectations of all healthcare professionals and clinical support staff, to deliver clinical and cost-effective services. The increasing age of the population is also increasing the demand and cost of healthcare in a service where resources are finite. The need to both perform and demonstrate evidence-based practice is now perceived as essential in order to provide the best outcomes for the least input.

A number of developments aimed at addressing these issues have taken place over the past decade:

- Since 1991, the NHS has attempted to identify and prioritize its research needs in a systematic way. A National Research and Development (R&D) Programme attempts to influence healthcare research using a 'bottom-up' approach, incorporating consumers' views and promoting the utilization of research into practice (DoH 1991).
- Enthusiasm from healthcare professionals to reflect, be critical of their practice and look for research evidence to provide the best possible treatment and care. This has led to the development of academic institutions, such as the Centre for Evidenced-Based Medicine Oxford, and the recent wealth of books and journal articles on both reflective and evidence-based practice.
- The development of centres, programmes, journals and databases to support the reviews of primary research and in some cases provide clear guidelines for interventions. For example: the NHS Centre for Reviews and Dissemination at the University of York; the Promoting Action on Clinical Effectiveness Kings Fund Programme (PACE); *Evidenced Based Nursing Journal*; and Medline/CINAHL electronic databases.
- Commitment from the current government to establish structures and systems in healthcare to promote clinical effectiveness and reduce variation in both professional practice and patient outcomes (DOH 1997, 1998; NHSE 1999). From April 1999, each healthcare organization will now be accountable for the clinical quality of care in addition to managing budgets, through the development of systems of clinical governance.

There is now a requirement to implement continuous quality improvements that may involve changes in treatment and care, in terms of practising in a different way, ceasing a particular intervention or using new resources, technology or skills. Whether or not improvements are made is often at the mercy of the clinician or manager's skill to:

- identify that a problem exists in practice
- find the evidence, demonstrating good practice or standards
- establish what should be done and who should be involved in making an improvement
- be creative in securing effective and efficient changes
- demonstrate improvement and share this with others.

This chapter is concerned with how best to demonstrate and secure the required resources or changes to make a sustained improvement in everyday practice, and how research evidence can and should ultimately influence policy, guidelines or protocol at local or national level.

Action point

- Have you ever had an idea about a change or innovation in your practice area that you have just not been able to achieve or implement?
- Does it all seem too much to contemplate at times?
- Spend some time thinking of ways that you might be able to make that important change.

The national context of research

The NHS R&D programme established in 1991 was the first attempt in Britain to establish a strategy for research, aiming to support the promotion of health and healthcare provision. Its main purpose was to identify research priorities in relation to health need and ensure that relevant research information was available to inform decisions on health policy, practice and the management of services (Jones et al. 1995). The programme has also evaluated methods of promoting implementation of research findings into healthcare (DoH 1995).

Over the past two years, two government white papers have outlined how the NHS will create new structures and systems to guarantee the highest quality care to all patients (DoH 1997, 1998). The provision of healthcare based on credible research evidence is one of the main elements proposed by the government, and a number of structures are to be developed to support clinicians and managers in its implementation.

Standards for services and clinical interventions are to be set at the highest level, defining what patients can expect to receive from the NHS:

- The National Institute for Clinical Excellence (NICE) will bring together work already performed by many professional organizations which receive DoH funding. Its purpose will be to identify new interventions from research findings, including those undertaken by the R&D programme, appraise the findings for clinical and cost-effectiveness, and provide and disseminate guidelines and supporting audit methodologies for implementation. It is anticipated that any gaps in research evidence will be addressed through the R&D programme.
- National Service Frameworks will set national standards and provide models for specific services or care groups, and develop performance indicators to enable progress to be measured. Included in the frameworks will be a review of the evidence base for diagnosis, treatment, therapy and care. Among the first frameworks to be produced were services for cancer, mental health and coronary heart disease.

Delivery of the standards will be through the following:

- A system of clinical governance whereby organizations are accountable for the quality of clinical treatments and care. This will require a number of existing services to develop formal links with each other to provide a co-ordinated organizational service for quality improvement.
- To meet the highest standards of care, all clinicians will have a responsibility to deliver evidence-based practice and be supported by their organization in the skills necessary. These include locating and interpreting research evidence, identifying achievable standards, clinical and cost-effective practice, and managing change. Decision-making in healthcare, either clinical

or managerial, should be informed by evidence of some quality to inform every stage of the healthcare process.

- The effectiveness of clinical interventions and the organization of teams and services against set standards will need to be measured through clinical and organizational audit. This will require a stronger research evidence-based approach in defining standards, guidelines and protocols and more creativity in developing new ways to practise. Research and development departments within trusts will play a role in co-ordinating research projects to address knowledge gaps in practice and services.
- Staff will be supported in their responsibility to keep up to date with the knowledge and skills required to perform in their role. There should be opportunities provided within the organization for professional support, such as having preceptorship programmes in place and a nominated clinical supervisor. There should also be opportunities for continued development such as formal education within and outside the trust, or the development of clinical, managerial, research, audit and teaching skills as part of the role of the healthcare professional.
- Staff performance will also need to be monitored through a variety of mechanisms, such as assessment of clinical competence, ability to meet agreed objectives and clinical outcome measures, if appropriate.
- Assessment and monitoring of clinical risk will be required within organizations. Action will need to be taken from reported untoward incidents and complaints.
- There has also been recognition that to achieve the highest-quality care, professionals will have to learn to work collaboratively, in multiprofessional teams, across purchaser/provider boundaries, and involve patients and health service users in improvements to provide patient-focused care.

Healthcare trusts will now be responsible for providing co-ordinated systems to guarantee high-quality clinical and cost-effective healthcare. In the new NHS, evidence from all types of research, will have a major influence on future healthcare decisions. Methods to assist the implementation of research, such as systematic reviews and Meta analysis, and the provision of guidance for good practice will undoubtedly enhance the use of research in practice.

Influencing policy makers

Previously in the NHS, development of policy tended to be based on personal values of the policy makers themselves or focused on achieving the agendas of services. Muir Gray (1998, p 71) describes three factors that influence decisions about policy:

- evidence of clinical and cost-effectiveness
- available resources
- values and beliefs of patients, the public or policy makers.

Bury (1998) suggests that policy decisions are driven by fashion, pragmatism and idealism. Changes may be made in practice due to pressures from a variety of sources without a sound evidence base, and the research that follows tries to substantiate its introduction.

If there is a drive in the NHS to provide evidenced-based clinical practice, there should be a commitment from policy makers to apply the same principles to decision making.

The raising awareness in the NHS over the past decade of limited resources and budgetary pressures has influenced the need to base healthcare policy on research evidence that has demonstrable positive outcomes.

Clinical effectiveness

Reviewing primary research by undertaking or using a systematic review on a topic or clinical intervention can be used to inform clinical guidelines. Clinical guidelines 'are systematically developed statements which assist clinicians and patients in making decisions about appropriate treatment for specific conditions' (NHSE 1996). Clinical guidelines have three key features:

- The guidelines are based on the best available evidence in that a systematic or rigorous process has been undertaken to evaluate and synthesize evidence of effectiveness.
- Guidelines deal with specific clinical interventions for specific patient populations.
- A systematic approach is taken as to who is to be involved in the guideline development, and will include the patient's perspective.

Guidelines will therefore be instrumental in informing policy decisions as a source of evidence and will make clear recommendations for practice. This evidence can then be used to make broader policy decisions, and an example will be discussed later.

Cost-effectiveness

Budgetary restrictions have driven the need to make a clearer distinction in policy development between the values of policy makers and a sound evidence base. In addition, there is now a requirement to analyse the benefits of treatment and care beyond clinical effectiveness alone (Muir Gray 1998). Cost-effectiveness therefore has an important role to play in making policy decisions by undertaking a form of economic evaluation, which compares two or more alternative interventions in terms of their costs and predicted outcomes.

Cost-effectiveness refers to having the best outcomes for the least input. A cost-effective intervention is one that 'gives a better or equivalent benefit, for lower or equivalent costs, or where the relative improvement in outcome is higher than the relative difference in cost' (Chambers 1998). An example of this may be the purchasing of a new cholesterol-measuring machine in the GP's surgery. An expensive machine, which has more features to measure different cholesterol factors, will cost significantly more than a basic one and thus use money that might be spent on other patient needs. However, if by having all these special features it can be demonstrated that fewer patients have a reduced risk of developing cardiovascular problems, these factors would be taken into account in making a decision about purchasing equipment.

In any policy decision, there is now a greater emphasis on cost-benefit analysis of the intervention. This is a technique where evidence of the costs and benefits of various interventions are analysed and translated into financial terms (Muir Gray 1998). Economic evaluation of interventions will influence policy making, and research in future may therefore have to consider beneficial outcomes in terms of cost if it is to impact on decision making.

Public and patient values

Values are concerned with what counts as fair in society or healthcare, and have a strong influence on policy decisions. Services and treatments are developed to meet the needs of service users who should have an opportunity to contribute to developments and changes in practice and policy.

Case study

A simple example of using research to influence policy in an acute trust, using an economic evaluation (the principles here could be applied to any area).

It was established through clinical audit that patients undergoing day surgery experienced moderate to severe pain during the first two days following discharge. The analgesia prescribed on the ward at the time of discharge was given to patients at the discretion of surgeons and anaesthetists. For those patients who did receive the analgesia, it was inadequate for many in terms of the amount of tablets prescribed and their ability to relieve pain. In addition, little information was given on how to manage pain at home. Patients contacted their GPs regularly for more analgesia, either through a consultation at the surgery or, in some cases, by requesting a home visit (Haddock et al. 1999).

Prescribing clinically effective analgesia to every patient, increasing the number of tablets prescribed and providing supporting information would increase the cost to the trust by approximately £1 per patient. However, a re-audit implementing the above demonstrated that GP consultation was significantly reduced and the analgesia provided increased pain relief. If this was adopted as a trust policy it would provide significant cost benefits and reduced morbidity, and thus increase clinical and cost-effectiveness. Initial costs would be offset by reducing costs in primary care and improving the patients' experience of pain. Clinical guidelines were then developed to implement a local prescribing protocol, which may influence the development of a trust policy for all day-surgery patients. A decision to introduce this as a policy within the trust would therefore have been informed by both an evidence base and a consideration of resources and patient care improvements.

Values would influence the decision to provide more analgesia, depending on the level of staff concern for patients' morbidity following discharge. Staff beliefs, along with the acute trust's beliefs regarding the responsibilities of the acute day-surgery service to provide medication for use when discharged, would also influence decisions to fund analgesia provision.

Using research to bid for resources or influence change

Health service managers have a responsibility to use the resources allocated to them to the best effect. When it has been identified that improvements can and should be made to existing practice, research evidence can be used in a variety of ways to influence change.

To set standards of good practice

If high standards have been achieved in other services, research evidence may have informed the type of intervention or organization of services provided to achieve them. For example, if research had demonstrated that patients who were assessed for pain levels following surgery using a trust-wide standardized pain assessment tool experience less pain by having regular analgesia, then a standard could be set that every patient will have their pain assessed postoperatively using a standardised assessment tool.

To ensure that a specific practice has been demonstrated to be clinically and cost-effective

Once realistic standards have been set, clinical guidelines can be developed to ensure that practice is consistent and will achieve the set standards. The main criteria for developing clinical guidelines are that they are based on research evidence or have been demonstrated to be an effective and efficient way to practise (NHSE 1996).

For example, when performing a relatively simple but essential assessment of a patient's temperature, the accuracy is dependent on where the thermometer is placed and how long it is in contact with the patient's body. A change in practice may occur if equipment other than a thermometer was used, for example to reduce the time required to read the result. This may require evidence to justify the introduction of the equipment and guidelines developed for its use.

To cease practice

If an intervention or the organization of a service is found to provide no identifiable benefit to the patient through the research process or clinical audit, then its continuation should be considered. Systematic reviews and Meta analysis may provide the best evidence to justify ceasing to perform a particular practice. Networking with wards or services in other healthcare trusts to establish whether or not it is practised gives a wider context to make a decision about whether to cease a practice.

A large element of risk taking is required both to change from one way of practising to another or to cease a practice. The use of research evidence provides a certain amount of security for staff and trusts making changes, however, the use of clinical audit to establish if improvements have been made will demonstrate whether practice meets the required standards.

Submitting proposals

When bidding for new resources or changes in practice, it is necessary to 'justify' to those who manage service budgets that resources should be allocated to particular aspects of care and treatment. To be successful, a good evidenced-based proposal must be developed to show that the benefits of changes are identified and understood by all the stakeholders involved. The following are essential elements that need to be included in any proposal for a change in practice.

Background to the change

This should include describing what the practice consists of, how it benefits the patient and why it needs to change. Include a local and national context and lead to the identification of the problem.

Review of the evidence

This should cover the search strategy for literature and include key search words, databases, Internet websites and the time period searched. The quality of the evidence should be summarized to show the type of evidence available:

- randomised control trial (RCT)
- systematic reviews of RCTs
- individual trials of inadequate size to detect adverse effects of treatment
- control trials without randomization
- observational studies
- reports of expert committees
- descriptive studies.

The literature review should be clear and supportive in terms of justifying a change in practice. If there is evidence that successful changes have occurred in another healthcare trust, this should be made explicit in the literature review and given an emphasis to show that change can be achieved.

Current practice

This should describe the main elements of current practice.

The proposed change or resources required

This should include the aim, objectives and any standards that should be achieved. There should be details of what is being proposed for change and what is required to improve practice. The magnitude of the benefit compared with current practice should be made explicit. Those who will be responsible for change should be identified as well as how the change will be implemented in practice. The change may require a piloting period with an evaluation of its effectiveness and identification any barriers. Timescales should be included, with a start date.

There should also be details relating to the new practice, identifying any changes in patient safety and increases in clinical risk, and increases in the cost of services. The cost to services, the directorate, other services/directorate or any other part of the NHS should be stated.

Costs will need to be up-to-date and detailed. If any other sources of funding have been identified, detailed descriptions should be given.

Evaluation

Evaluation tools and methods will need to be described with estimated timescales.

Implementing change

Once an evidence base, and perhaps a baseline audit, has been undertaken and it has been identified that a change in practice is required, clinical guidelines may be developed to guide clinicians and standardize practice to reduce variation.

The Kings Fund programme relating to promoting action on clinical effectiveness (PACE) has undertaken 16 different projects. The programme has identified and reported on the immense difficulties in the management and implementation processes involved in implementing research findings into practice and NHS services. A report on the progress and lessons learned from the project has illustrated a number of key components identified from the project in the management of change, involving all healthcare professionals (Dunning et al. 1999). The authors have provided honest reports of progress and the real issues encountered, concluding that change:

* is a messy business, requiring facilitation, flexibility and project leaders able to coax, cajole and drive the work forward
* is not a linear task but a group of complex and inter-related tasks
* takes time, usually far longer than expected
* is expensive, requiring lots of commitment if success is to be achieved.

Ten essential tasks have been identified as critical in the management of change when undertaking projects to improve clinical effectiveness. The project to improve patients' experiences of pain following discharge from day surgery was undertaken at the Royal Hospital in Chesterfield (Haddock et al. 1999), and will be used to illustrate how each task was achieved.

1. Choosing where to start

Ensure that there is local support for the proposal for change
Current literature on post-discharge pain following day surgery was scarce and evidence of pain management in day surgery provided conflicting guidelines. The pain department within the trust had raised the profile of pain control for inpatients. Pain management was therefore an important area for the day surgery unit to address and was a priority in the trust. Patients' experiences of pain following discharge from day surgery, the analgesia prescribed and their contacts with primary care were assessed in the first stage of the audit cycle.

2. Engaging clinicians

Securing support from clinical staff
The project was fully supported by the clinical director and the department of pain management. Stakeholders in day surgery, pain management, anaesthetics, pharmacy, clinical audit and day surgery nursing and management were identified and consulted about the project.

3. Involving patients

Be clear about why patients need to be involved and how to do so
Patients were assessed for their pain levels for two days after discharge and whether there had been cause to contact their GP or district nurse. They were asked to complete a questionnaire and given an opportunity to comment on the quality of their care on the day surgery unit. As a result of their comments, a comprehensive patient information leaflet was developed regarding the administration of analgesia provided on discharge and general pain management.

4. Defining local standards

Agree locally intended standards of practice
Standards of care and the maximum amount of pain that patients should expect to experience, and the effectiveness of their analgesia, was identified from the literature and modified following consultation with all stakeholders. Clinically and cost-effective forms of analgesia were identified using systematic reviews and a standardized prescribing protocol for everyday surgery patients was produced. Patients were assessed for sensitivities and the anaesthetists or surgeons prescribed one of two possible options of analgesia packs. Each pack contained an appropriate patient information leaflet.

5. Keeping in touch

Keep the stakeholders and those with direct interest in the project informed on progress
To enable the work to be taken forward, stakeholders in the project were updated regularly on the progress of the project. Following the initial audit, the results were presented to surgery and anaesthetic audit meetings, and the original stakeholders.

6. Securing change

Ensure that change is realistic and secured
The results of the initial audit demonstrated that standards were not met and patients were receiving analgesia inconsistently on the judgement of individual doctors. Patients experienced excessive pain and were not provided with an adequate amount or strength of analgesia. Relief of pain following administration of analgesia was also poor.

The consultant in pain management presented the protocol to all the prescribers in day surgery for consultation, comments and to justify the choice of analgesia. Arrangements were made with pharmacy to allow analgesia packs to be ward-dispensed by nursing staff. This would improve the efficiency of the discharge process for both staff and patients. All the ward nurses had been involved in the development of the patient information leaflet and were able to educate patients effectively using the leaflet as a guide.

7. Providing services

Ensure that services can be provided to match the proposed change in practice
The project secured an increase in resources from the district health authority to pump-prime the costs of the analgesia packs. An assessment of the resource consequences of the initiative was performed and the re-audit was scheduled to be finished in time for the next round of contacts with purchasers. The results were then provided with evidence of cost consequences for the trust and the demonstrable improvements in services for day-surgery patients.

The project also demonstrated that pain relief could be improved and there was a guarantee that patients could be treated on a day-case basis and have their pain managed to the same degree as if they were an inpatient. This had implications at the time for waiting list initiatives driven by government policy.

8. Measuring impact

Establish if improvements have been made
A re-audit of patients' experiences was undertaken following the change in practice. The results were compared with the initial audit and the standards set by the relevant staff. There was a significant improvement in patients' experiences and a reduction in primary

care contact. Ward dispensing of analgesia reduced time spent by nurses attending pharmacy.

9. Sustaining change

Ensure that change becomes routine practice

Disseminating success of the project is important in securing any resources required to sustain the change. A decision was made within the directorate to recurrently fund the analgesia packs and take responsibility to provide patients with analgesia for up to four days following discharge, since cost savings were made by reducing primary care contact.

Documentation in the form of nursing assessment for sensitivities and the prescribing protocol was then incorporated into current documentation. The prescribing protocol was introduced at junior doctors' induction programmes. Training packages, including arrangements for ward dispensing and guidelines to give patient information using the leaflets, were produced for new nursing staff.

10. Learning lessons

Reflect on the experience of the project and learn lessons for the next project

Lessons were learned at each stage of the process of implementing change, and subsequent practice was modified. This included the following.

- Setting standards too high and negotiating with staff to lower them.
- Despite at least five pilots the audit tool needed required further changes to elicit more detailed information.
- The documentation and dispensing of the ward packs generated teething problems which could not have been foreseen, for example patients written up for wrong packs and the documentation for ward dispensing requiring more information than originally thought.
- Piloting, evaluating and amending the patient information leaflet at least four times, with subsequent reprinting. This process is ongoing to incorporate patients' comments or requests for more information.

Further issues that required evaluation were also addressed and the process of establishing effectiveness and improving patients' experiences and staff efficiency continues.

Action point

- Reconsider an innovation that you wanted to implement, make a detailed plan outlining the key issues that you must consider in preparing for your change.
- Do you have any new ideas that you might use after reading this chapter?
- Are you going to have a go now?

Conclusion

There is a new impetus within the NHS to support professionals in the provision of healthcare interventions that have been demonstrated to be clinically and cost-effective at all stages during assessment, diagnosis, treatment and care. The need to commission, report and disseminate high-quality research in a systematic way has therefore never been greater. Prescriptive research will increasingly be expected to consider the cost and efficiency of an intervention, in addition to its clinical effectiveness, so that service managers can make informed decisions to develop local policy and guidelines, and improve clinical practice.

Research evidence can then be utilized in practice to inform decision making and act as a lever for change. High-quality research is often scarce for many practices, however, even where there is an abundance of clear, unequivocal evidence, the process of change is usually prolonged and problematic. It requires, among other things, commitment, support, sophisticated communication skills and, from the practitioner's point of view, endless patience.

References and further reading

Bury T (1998) Getting research into practice. In Bury TJ, Mead JM (eds) Evidence Based Healthcare. A practical guide for therapists, chapter 4. Oxford: Butterworth-Heinmann.
Chambers R (1998) Clinical Effectiveness Made Easy. Oxford: Radcliffe Medical Press.

Department of Health (1991) Research for Health: a research and development strategy for the NHS. London: The Stationery Office.

Department of Health (1995) Methods for the Implementation of Findings of Research. Priorities for Evaluation. Advisory group to the NHS Central R&D Committee. Leeds: Department of Health.

Department of Health (1997) The New NHS: modern, dependable. London: The Stationery Office.

Department of Health (1998) A First Class Service: quality in the new NHS. London: The Stationery Office.

Dunning M, Abi-Aad G, Gilbert D, Hutton H, Brown C (1999) Experience, Evidence and Everyday Practice. London: Kings Fund.

Godlee F (1998) Applying research evidence to individual patients (Editorial). British Medical Journal 316: 1621-2.

Haddock J, Challands A, Stevens J, Wong C, Walters S (1999) Patient controlled oral analgesia at home (PCOAH) for the management of post-discharge pain following day surgery. Journal of One Day Surgery 8 (4): 3-8.

Jones R, Lamont R, Haines A (1995) Setting priorities for research and development in the NHS: a case study on the interface between primary and secondary care. British Medical Journal 311: 1080-2.

Muir Gray J (1997) Evidenced Based Health Care. London: Churchill Livingstone.

Muir Gray J (1998) Evidence based policy making. In Haines A, Donald A (eds) Getting Research into Practice, chapter 9. London: BMJ Publishing Group.

NHSE (1996) Clinical Guidelines. Using clinical guidelines to improve patient care within the NHS. Leeds: NHS Executive.

NHSE (1999) Clinical Governance Quality in the NHS. Leeds: NHS Executive.

Index